Leila Azouaou

Hereditary diseases Clinical cases

Leila Azouaou

Hereditary diseases Clinical cases

Renal metabolic and overload diseases

ScienciaScripts

Imprint

Cover image: www.ingimage.com

This book is a translation from the original published under ISBN 978-620-6-69844-9.

Publisher:
Sciencia Scripts
is a trademark of
Dodo Books Indian Ocean Ltd. and OmniScriptum S.R.L publishing group

120 High Road, East Finchley, London, N2 9ED, United Kingdom
Str. Armeneasca 28/1, office 1, Chisinau MD-2012, Republic of Moldova, Europe
Printed at: see last page
ISBN: 978-620-8-26043-9

FOREWORD

This Manual has been designed as an aid for nephrology students. Its aim is to help them understand the mechanisms underlying the disease and its consequences. It provides a general overview of current information on hereditary kidney diseases, with particular emphasis on the diagnosis and management of hereditary overload renal disease and metabolic disease. The expected results offer hope of further progress in the future.

CONTENTS

INTRODUCTION

Rare kidney diseases can be broken down into three groups conditions :

• **congenital anomalies in renal development**,

• **identified monogenetic kidney diseases**,

• **nephrotic syndromes**.

These diseases have in common a rare incidence, a phenotypic presentation that varies according to age, a risk of progression to renal failure, hypertension and possible repercussions on growth in children.

All of these rare diseases require early and appropriate treatment to slow their progression, as well as prolonged follow-up, for many of them throughout adult life... They can be broken down into **two groups of disorders**: congenital and hereditary.

1st group - congenital anomalies in renal development

They are characterised by malformed kidneys (renal dysplasia) or smaller kidneys (hypoplasia). These anomalies may be strictly isolated, or sometimes associated with urinary or extra-renal malformations. They may be asymptomatic, and many are detected by antenatal ultrasound. They may have a variety of causes, including genetic, environmental or uncertain.

2nd group - monogenic hereditary kidney diseases identified

They can affect any structure of the nephron and require specific early treatment:

• **Tubulopathies**: Bartter's syndrome, Gitelman's syndrome, Lowe's syndrome, Fanconi's syndrome, Dent's syndrome, Hypouricemia, Acidosis, Hypophosphatemic rickets, Cystinosis, etc.

• **Cystic diseases**: cystic dystrophy, recessive polycystic kidney disease, dominant childhood polycystic kidney disease, sclerosis, Bourneville's tuberous disease, von Hippel-Lindau disease, glomerulocystic syndromes, etc.

• **Tubulointerstitial diseases**: nephronophthisis, BOR and Bardet-Biedl syndrome, familial hyperuricemia, cystic renal medullary disease.

• **Glomerular diseases** : Alport syndrome, osteo-onycho-dysplasia, hereditary cortico-resistant nephrotic syndrome (NS), Finnish NS, autosomal dominant focal glomerulosclerosis, autosomal recessive cortico-resistant NS, Denys-Drash syndrome, Frasier syndrome, autosomal recessive diffuse mesangial sclerosis, Pierson syndrome, Chimke syndrome, Galloway syndrome, familial benign haematuria, etc.

• **Metabolic lithiasis**: oxalosis, cystinuria-lysinuria, idiopathic hypercalciuria...

• Certain **kidney tumours, hereditary or not** (Wilms)3rd group - nephrotic syndromes

These include idiopathic nephrosis and other idiopathic chronic glomerulopathies (extra-membranous glomerulonephritis or glomerulonephritis caused by foetal alloimmunisation, etc.).

I-A FEW GENETIC FACTS

The first cell of the embryo contains all the genetic information that will enable it to manufacture the elements that each cell needs throughout its life. In the cell, the genetic material takes the form of filaments, or chromosomes, that can be observed under the microscope.

What is a chromosome?

The somatic cells of a human organism contain 46 chromosomes in their nucleus, divided into 23 pairs. Each pair consists of one copy of the chromosome inherited from the father and one copy of the chromosome inherited from the mother.

There are 22 pairs of chromosomes, identical in both sexes, called autosomes; they are numbered from 1 to 22.

The 23rd pair consists of two so-called sex chromosomes. They are essential for sex determination and are different in women and men. In women, pair 23 is formed by an X chromosome from the mother and a different chromosome, the Y chromosome, from the father.

Only the nuclei of sexual reproductive cells (ova in women, spermatozoa in men) have a single copy of each pair of chromosomes and contain 23 chromosomes. The fertilised egg, the result of the union of the egg and the spermatozoon, contains the genetic material of both parents. This first cell multiplies to form the several billion cells that make up a human being.

How is gender determined?

The sex chromosomes are distributed randomly in the sex cells. In women , the ovum contains one of the two X chromosomes . In men, the sperm contains the X or Y chromosome.

If the first cell of the embryo contains two X chromosomes (one from the mother, the other from the father), the embryo becomes a girl. If this first cell contains one X chromosome (from the mother) and one Y chromosome (from the father), the embryo becomes a boy.

What is a gene?

It is the elementary unit of the genetic heritage of all living beings. The set of genes determines both the characteristics common to all members of a species and the characteristics specific to each individual. It is estimated that humans have 30,000 different genes.
Genes are located on chromosomes and are made up of a molecule called deoxyribonucleic acid (DNA) on which bases follow one another in a precise order.
A gene is a region of DNA that codes, or in other words directs, the production of one or more proteins. Proteins can be seen as the machine tools that make the body function. But **this** operation is complicated. The expression of a gene varies over time and varies from one organ to another. In addition, proteins interact with each other and their interactions change over time.
Each protein is made up of amino acids in a precise order. It is the normal succession of groups of three bases on the gene that determines the normal suction of amino acids in the protein. corresponding protein, ensuring that it functions properly.

What is a mutation?

This is a sudden chemical change in the gene sequence resulting in a change in the information encoded by the gene: the modified gene is said to be a mutated gene. This change in information can be passed on to the offspring of an affected person. Mutations are responsible for the evolution of species. Their causes are not well known. For a given hereditary disease, the position of the mutation in the gene and/or the type of gene alteration vary.
Depending on its position in the gene or its type, a mutation may be responsible for

- The absence of the protein normally codes for the gene ;
- Or the manufacture of a defective protein that works badly.

The position of the mutation in the gene and/or its type may vary from one family to another. But all the members of a family, if they are affected, have the same mutation.

II- ORGANIGRAMME OF NEPHROPATHIES, DISEASES "HEREDITARY" METABOLIC DISEASES, OVERLOAD DISEASES

1- Glomerular nephropathy and "hereditary" metabolic diseases, overload diseases

- Lysosomal diseases:
- Fabry
- Left-handed
- Nephrosialidosis
- Others (Hurler, gangliosidosis, sphingolipidosis)

- Diabetes
- Amyloidosis
- Familial lecithin-cholesterol acyl transferase deficiency
- Lipoprotein glomerulopathy

2- Tubulointerstitial nephropathy and 'hereditary' metabolic diseases
overload

- Glycogenosis
- Cystinosis
- Tyrosinosis
- Oxalose

Clinical cases

The patient was 37 years old, and was found to have end-stage CKD by chance. On investigation, cardiac symptoms were found, associated with t h e presence of a left ventricular hypertrophy; skin : brown spots on the thighs with endocrine disorders such as hypothyroidism; brain MRI: no abnormalities; The enzymatic study of the dosage of a galactosidase is collapsed while the dosage of lyso GL3 is high, the genetic study finds a heterozygous mutation c 779G> A (p.Gly260Glu) All the other members were explored and the same genetic mutation was found including a 5 year old male child, a brother and two women from the same family (mother and sister) who are ill.

Question 1: What type of genetic disease?

The patient was a 3-year-old child who presented to the emergency department with convulsions in a febrile state following a recurrent urinary tract infection associated with vomiting and dehydration.
At the labstix: haematuria: ++.

Renal ultrasound: nephrocalcinosis Renal work-up: end-stage CKD.
ECG: heart rhythm disorder

AGT activity assay: collapsed AGXT gene mutation
Q1: What type of genetic disease
Clinical case 3

The patient was a 3-year-old child who presented to withconvulsions in a febrile emergency following a recurrent urinary tract infection associated with vomiting and dehydration.
At the labstix: haematuria: ++.

Renal ultrasound: nephrocalcinosis Renal work-up: end-stage CKD.
ECG: heart rhythm disorder

AGT activity assay: collapsed AGXT gene mutation
Q1: What type of genetic disease?

III-GLOMERULAR NEPHROPATHY AND "HEREDITARY" DISEASES METABOLISM, OVERLOAD DISEASES

1- Lysosomal disease

The body is made up of several billion cells. Each cell is bounded by a membrane that surrounds the cytoplasm, which contains the nucleus and several different structures, including lysosomes. These are essential for the body to function properly [1]. Lysosomes are small formations, also bounded by a membrane. They are the cleaning sites of the cell. In fact, it is in the lysosomes that the substances transported there are cut up into pieces. Remember that this destruction is part of the normal process of life and that living matter is in a perpetual state of renewal. When the lysosomes are not functioning, this cleaning process is no longer guaranteed: the undegraded molecules accumulate and disrupt the functions of the cells [2].

Clinical cases 1

The patient was 37 years old and was found to have end-stage CKD by chance. On investigation, cardiac symptoms were found, associated with the presence of left ventricular hypertrophy; The enzymatic study of the dosage of a galactosidase is collapsed while the dosage of lyso GL3 is high, the genetic study finds a heterozygous mutation c 779G> A (p.Gly260Glu) All the other members were explored and the same genetic mutation was found including a 5 year old male child, a brother and two women from the same family (mother and sister) who are ill.

Question 1: What type of genetic disease?

A-Fabry disease is a rare disease; according to studies, its frequency is estimated to be between 1 in 40,000 and 1 in 100,000 [3]. It occurs in all countries and was first diagnosed in 1898 by two dermatologists. Johannes Fabry (in Germany) and William Anderson (in England) each reported, independently of the other, the first descriptions of the disease[4] .

Numerous patient observations.

Numerous observations of patients have subsequently made it possible to describe various clinical aspects and to gradually understand that :

- The disease is characterised by the accumulation of abnormal lipid material in the body's cells.

- This material accumulates in lysosomes, which are special structures in the body. of the cell

- This accumulation is due to a deficiency in an enzyme present in the lysosome, a-galactosidase A

- The disease is hereditary, with transmission within families linked to the X chromosome.

1- Definition :Fabry disease is a disease of the lysosomes.

the body is made up of several billion cells. Each cell consists of cytoplasm bounded by a membrane. In the cytoplasm, there is a nucleus (containing the chromosomes) and several different structures, including the lysosomes, which are essential for the organism to function properly. Lysosomes are small membrane-bound formations. They are the cell's recycling sites. In fact, it is in the lysosomes that substances are cut up and transported. Remember that this destruction is part of the normal process of life and that living matter is constantly being renewed. When the lysosomes are not functioning, this recycling is no longer ensured: the undegraded molecules accumulate and disrupt the functions of the cells [5].

What happens in Fabry disease?

The disease results from the abnormal deposition in the cells of a glycosphingolipid substance, globotriaosylceramide (abbreviated to Gb3; GL3), also known as ceramide trihexoside. The primary defect responsible is a deficiency in a-galactosidase A, the enzyme which normally degrades GL3 . This major discovery in the 1960s made it possible to diagnose the disease by measuring a-galctosidase A activity in the blood of boys [6].

Techniques enabling large quantities of human a- galctosidase A to be produced by genetic engineering have stimulated research leading to the development of enzyme replacement therapy, opening up a new era in the treatment of Fabry disease. This treatment is now combined with symptomatic treatment [7].

The transmission of Fabry disease within families

Studies of patients' families had long suggested that transmission was X-linked recessive **Criteria for recognition of the disease in families**

- **The disease appears in boys**

- **Women may have no signs at all, or they may present with a**

usually less severe than in men.

- **A man ill has no son sick, but transmits the gene anomaly to her daughters.**
- **An affected woman can pass on the gene anomaly to her sons**

and girls.

It was in 1986 that the gene coding for a-galactosidase A , located on the X chrosome , was identified and named GLA . This discovery paved the way for molecular studies to identify mutations in the gene in patients. More than two hundred mutations in the GLA gene have been characterised, most of which are unique to each family [8].

.

A few essential definitions?

If the GLA gene mutation is found on :

- **A man's unique X chromosome is said to be sick hemizygote :**

- **One of a woman's 2 X chromosomes, the woman is said to have carrier of the mutation is heterozygous or a carrier.**

- **The woman's 2 X chromosomes are said to be homozygous.**

What is the risk of transmitting the disease to children?

The risk of transmission of the disease from parents to children depends on the type of union . three types of union are possible .

1- **Union of a heterozygous woman with a healthy man** .

In this mother, one of the X chromosomes carries the mutated gene and the other carries the normal gene. With each pregnancy, each boy has a 1 in 2 risk of being ill and each girl a 1 in 2 risk of being heterozygous carrier.
Genetically unaffected boys and girls can be reassured for themselves and their offspring [9].

2- Union of a sick haemizygous man and a healthy woman In this man, the X chromosome carries the mutated gene. All the girls receive this X chromosome; they are heterozygous and risk passing on the anomaly, generally to some of their children. The boys receive the Y chromosome from their father; all are unaffected.

3- Union of aman hemizygous ill and a woman heterozygous

This situation is exceptional, except in cases of consanguinity. This is the the only situation in which a homozygous daughter could be born ill his 2 X chromosomes carry the mutated gene.

4- An exceptional location

The disease follows in a boy whose mother is not a carrier of the mutation, known as neomutation, occurred suddenly during fertilisation. As explained above, this boy risks transmitting the mutation to the girls.

The disease can appear in different clinical forms:

The accumulation of clinical observations and their comparison with the results of biological and/or gene diagnostics have made it possible to distinguish different clinical aspects:

- Complete a-galactosidase A deficiency and the resulting accumulation of abnormal GL3 deposits are responsible for the clinical manifestations (pain, skin, eye, kidney, etc.).

) observed in haemizygous men with the classic form of Fabry disease [10][.

- It was traditionally thought that heterozygous women with the mutation showed few or no symptoms. We now know that many of these women do have symptoms, and that the disease is later-onset and more moderate than in men. However, it can present with the same severity.
- Some doctors have reported atypical observations characterised by late cardiac involvement in haemizygous men with residual a-galactosidase A activity.
- Others have reported atypical observations characterised by apparently isolated renal involvement (a clinical form known as renal variant) [11] .

How to explain clinical variability in women

To compensate for the fact that boys (XY) have a single set of genes located on the X chromosome compared to girls (XX), a complex and as yet unresolved mechanism, the inactivation of the X chromosome, is established in girls.

This mechanism has 3 points:

-In a woman's somatic cells, only one X chromosome is active. The second X chromosome remains condensed and therefore inactive, which means that the gene products of this chromosome cannot be produced.

-inactivation of the X chromosome occurs very early in embryonic life (between 3 days and the end of the first week of development).

-In each cell, the inactivated X chromosome may be of paternal or maternal origin; in a given cell, the inactivation of one of these two chromosomes is entirely random. But once established, the inactivation is permanent and is transmitted stably and irreversibly to the daughter cells during cell division. When both X chromosomes are normal, either one or the other, the protein produced is normal. But the situation changes if one of the two chromosomes carries a mutated gene. This leads to cellular mosaicism, with variable proportions of cells in which the normal or abnormal gene is active. Inactivation of the X chromosome leads to this clinical variability, which ranges from minor manifestations to full expression of the disease and can be seen from one woman to another, and even in women from the same family [12].

The accumulation of GL3

GL3 can accumulate in the lysosomes of most cells that make up tissues, mainly in :

- Blood vessels throughout thebody endothelial and smooth muscle cells).
- The eye in the cornea (in the epithelial cells)
- The heart (in the muscle cells)
- The autonomic nervous system (in the ganglion cells)

What are the consequences of this accumulation in the cells?

The cells in which glycolipids accumulate in the lysosomes are large and have an abnormally clear appearance under light microscopy. Special stains on a previously frozen sample make it possible to confirm that these deposits are glycolipids. Finally, electron microscopy shows that these deposits correspond to dense, laminated inclusions with a striated appearance. They are bounded by a simple membrane. In hemizygous men with the classic form, these deposits are found in all tissues. In the renal glomerulus, for example, this accumulation of deposits is diffuseaffects all cells at an early stage a n d probably increases with age. In heterozygous women with the mutation, the accumulation of deposits only affects a certain number of cells [14].

2- Clinical :

a- Clinical abnormalities in haemizygous boys 1- Renal abnormalities
Abnormalities in tubular function

the tubular cells are altered during Fabry as a result of deposits, leading to nocturnal polyuria.

Proteinuria

It corresponds to the presence of proteinuria preceded by microalbuminuria, and appears between the ages of 20 and 30, sometimes before the age of 10. It remains moderate and rarely develops into a nephrotic syndrome.

Microscopic haematuria :

It occurs in a third of sick haemizygous men and is associated with proteinuria.

The Maltese crosses

Urine may contain glycolipid-laden tubular cells that have detached from the tubule wall. These cells take on a characteristic Maltese cross appearance when urine is observed under light microscopy and polarisation.

Renal failure

All haemizygous men with the classic form are at risk of developing kidney failure during their lifetime. It usually appears around the age of 30, sometimes before the age of 20. The rate of progression varies from one patient to another.

High blood pressure

It occurs in less than half of men. Blood pressure should be monitored in all men with fabry.

2- Cardiac disease in hemizygous men :

The preferential location of GL3 deposits determines the main cardiac manifestations.
Where the depots are located

- In cardiac muscle cells.

- In heart valves, especially aortic and mitral valves.

- In the cords of the mitral valve.

- In all intra-cardiac conduction nerve tissue.

- In the endothelial cells lining the vessels of the heart .

The greatest accumulation of deposits is in the left ventricle and mitral valve. Consequently, left ventricular hypertrophy, damage to the heart valves and conductance disorders are the most common and often the earliest manifestations of Fabry disease[15].

Left ventricular hypertrophy

This is one of the most common manifestations of Fabry disease, and is secondary to the accumulation of GL3 in cardiac muscle cells. This accumulation begins in the first few months of foetal life and continues throughout life.

Damage to the heart valves:

Involvement of the mitral valve

Mitral insufficiency is the most common type of valve damage. It is expressed by the discovery of a murmur that appeared in childhood or adolescence.

Damage to the aortic valve

It is less common. It usually represents a moderate form of aortic stenosis. Diagnosis is based on auscultation, which reveals an abnormal murmur, and echo-doppler.

Coronary complications :

- Stress angina pectoris

- Myocardial infarction.

Cardiac conduction disorders :

Cardiac rhythm disorders occur when the electrical excitation originates elsewhere than in the sinus node or when the electrical wave no longer follows the normal propagation pathways. infiltration of the conduction pathways by deposits can alter cardiac conduction.

3- Neurological damage: Cerebrovascular accidents :

They may occur in young adult men, but may be delayed. The clinical manifestations vary in severity: nausea or vomiting, double vision, balance problems, dizziness with shaky walking, sometimes paralysis of an arm, a leg or one side of the body (hemiplegia). These accidents may be transient (they regress) or permanent (they do not regress). They are due to damage to the brain, most frequently to the posterior part.

4- Pain

Pain is present in almost 90% of hemizygous boys with the classic form. We know that small nerve fibres are affected, in particular those that give the brain information about sensations on contact with hot or cold.

Acroparesthesia

These are tingling, pins and needles, persistent burns, and/or intense pain, such as stabbing, electric shocks, sometimes described as excruciating. Their intensity, when the diagnosis has not yet been made, can lead to the child being admitted to hospital as an emergency. These pains occur in the hands and feet, radiating to the forearms and arms, and thighs. They appear in boys, usually during childhood. between the ages of 3 and 12, sometimes during adolescence and more rarely after the age of 16. They can occur in attacks more or less spaced, more or less long, lasting from a few minutes to a few hours, even a few hours. days, giving way and sometimes leaving a permanent, less severe pain base.

5- Sweat abnormality

They are caused by damage to the small nerve fibres responsible for sweating or damage to the sweat glands. The disorders are noted from early childhood. The child does not sweat (anhidrosis) or more often, sweats little (hypohidrosis). These sweating anomalies are responsible for heat intolerance; this intolerance is marked by fever, respiratory discomfort and nausea. This can lead to heatstroke, vomiting and possibly loss of consciousness. At the very least, the child needs to be cooled down and rehydrated. Heat intolerance leads to intolerance to physical exertion. These disorders can be accompanied by a reduction in production tears or saliva .

6- **Angiokeratomas**

These are small skin lesions that appear in boys, generally in adolescence, around the age of 16, sometimes earlier, generally after acroparesthesia. They are characteristic of Fabry disease, and correspond to dilatations of the blood capillaries located in the superficial dermis. However, some men with the classic form of the disease do not never develop angikeratomas. Angiokeratomas are initially punctiform, ranging from dark red to dark blue, do not blanch on pressure, are flat or raised, and are usually hyperkeratotic. They can be found on the abdomen around the umbilicus, the hips buttocks, lower back, thighs, external genitalia. They are often symmetrical and rarely affect the face. Their number varies from patient to patient. Sometimes they are rare, isolated, sometimes affecting the fingertips, or found by careful examination of the skin around the genitals or umbilicus. Sometimes they are numerous, grouped over large areas of the body, and their size and/or number may increase with age.

7- **Digestive disorders**

These disorders are common and can occur as early as childhood. They are caused by deposits in the intestinal cells and nerves of the autonomic nervous system. Nausea, vomiting, a feeling of a distended abdomen and discomfort after meals can lead to a fear of certain foods and be responsible for frequent underweight or weight loss. Digestive bleeding may occur, leading to diagnostic errors. Painful abdominal attacks may simulate appendicitis or nephritic colic, leading to investigations of the digestive or urinary tract and sometimes to surgery.

8- Dizziness and reduced hearing Vertigo

They are due to damage to the vestibule. Severe vertigo can occur in adolescence and persist into adulthood. They may last for several days, or recur frequently, or give way to a feeling of permanent instability. They may be associated with nausea, vomiting or ringing in the ears.

Reduced hearing

hearing impairment is due to damage to the inner ear and is frequently associated with vestibular damage. Hearing impairment may be apparent or detected by an audiogram. Hearing monitoring is based on the audiogram, which enables the hearing loss to be quantified from one examination to the next.
Sudden onset of deafness is a medical emergency.

9- Fatigue

Painful attacks, intolerance to exertion and intolerance to heat are frequently accompanied by severe fatigue. The patient learns to save energy.

10- Lung disorders :

Pulmonary damage has been described in young non-smoking men. The lung damage resembles bronchitis associated with sputum and cough, which justifies stopping smoking.

11- Lymphedema

Oedema of the legs due to poor lymph circulation.

12- Ocular involvement

does the eye often suffer from fabry's disease? highly variable .

corneal deposits

These deposits can sometimes appear in children. They are very discreet give the cornea a cloudy appearance. Over time, the cornea takes on a very characteristic swirling appearance, with the cornea taking on a ground-glass appearance.

Lens opacities

These opacities form white lines crossing the posterior part of the lens.

At an advanced stage, they may be responsible for opacification of the crystalline; this is the wheel radius character.

Other anomalies

Dilatation of vessels in the conjunctiva or retina is also observed, but has no clinical consequences.

- 13 Atypical forms in hemizygous men: The cardiac variant :

This form has been described in men aged 40 or over, with residual a-galactosidase A activity and therefore without any of the classic signs of Fabry disease. These men misleadingly present as having isolated cardiac disease, specifically left ventricular hypertrophy, which poses numerous diagnostic problems.

Renal variant :

Some men present with severe isolated renal failure, most of whom are on dialysis, when Fabry disease is diagnosed. The diagnosis is often only made when characteristic deposits are found on a kidney biopsy.

b- Manifestations in heterozygous girls/women Clinical manifestations

For a long time, it was thought that girls did not suffer from Fabry disease. However, it was known that 70-80% of them developed corneal deposits in adulthood. In fact, pain in the extremities can occur during childhood or adolescence in many girls. These pains are sometimes not very sharp, but can be as intense as in boys.

Similarly, these girls may experience reduced sweating, intolerance to exertion and heat, febrile seizures, abdominal pain, digestive problems such as vomiting and diarrhoea, dizziness, tinnitus, fatigue, shortness of breath, lymphoedema and other symptoms that compromise their normal life.

If there is a family history, any of these symptoms should raise the diagnosis. The clinical examination must be careful to look for angiokeratomas which, if they exist, are often small in number. Some women develop cardiovascular complications, strokes and, more rarely, kidney complications comparable to those seen in haemizygous men. The organ most often affected is the heart, which may result in an increase in the thickness of the heart walls (left ventricular hypertrophy). After the age of 50 or 60, a conduction disorder between the atrium and the ventricle may appear, necessitating the fitting of a pacemaker. Heart failure is rare. Rarely, kidney damage occurs in adulthood [16].

3- Histological lesions Light microscopy :

The lesions of sphingolipid accumulation are visible on sections from the fixed paraffin-embedded biopsy. In glomeruli This overload is present in podocytes: they are voluminous and their cytoplasm is invaded by microvacuoles, giving them a honeycombed appearance. "honeycomb". On sections taken from the sample included in Under paraffin, these vacuoles are empty with the different stains. At high magnification, the inclusions are of variable size, empty or dense. This overload is found in the epithelial cells of Bowman's capsule; it is more difficult to recognise in the mesangial and endocapillary cells.

Other lesions may be added: thickening of the mesangial matrix with or without mesangial cell proliferation, fibrohyaline segmental lesions and progression to global sclerosis.

At the tubular level, the overload is very significant in the distal tubes, whereas the proximal tubes are usually normal. In the vessels**, the muscle cells and the endothelial cells contain vacuoles,** but hyaline balls are also sometimes visible in the muscle cells. Damage to the endothelial cells of the peritubular capillaries is important to assess for the follow-up of gene therapy [17].

Immunofluorescence: immunofluorescence is often negative. It may reveal non-specific glomerular segmental IGM deposits and vascular C3 deposits[18].

Electron microscopy :

All glomerular cells contain abnormal dense inclusions. These inclusions vary in size and shape. They are usually bounded by a simple membrane. They can take on different appearances: either a totally compact appearance, or a laminated appearance with regular alternation of light and dark bands, more often a concentric onion bulb structure, with lamellae of irregular thickness constituting the myelin bodies, or a complex organisation of dense laminae. These inclusions are very numerous in podocytes or large inclusions often pushing back the nucleus. They are less abundant in in other glomerular cells . They are less abundant in other glomerular cells. They are found in large numbers in distal tubular cells, and discreetly in proximal cells. In vessels, they are present in all endothelial and smooth muscle cells [19].

a- Haemizygous men

Overload lesions in males:

– All glomerular cells

– All vascular and interstitial cells

– Certain cells in the distal tubules

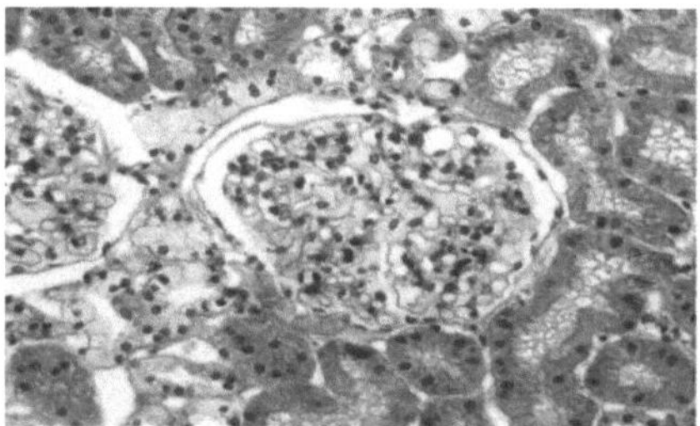

Figure 1: Fabry lesions [20].

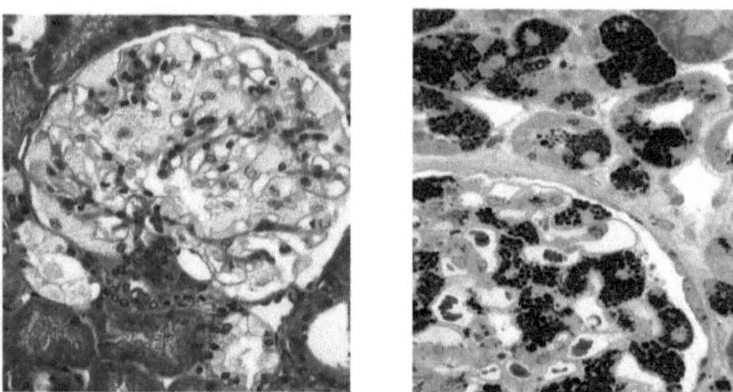

Figure 2: Glomerular overload lesions . [21]

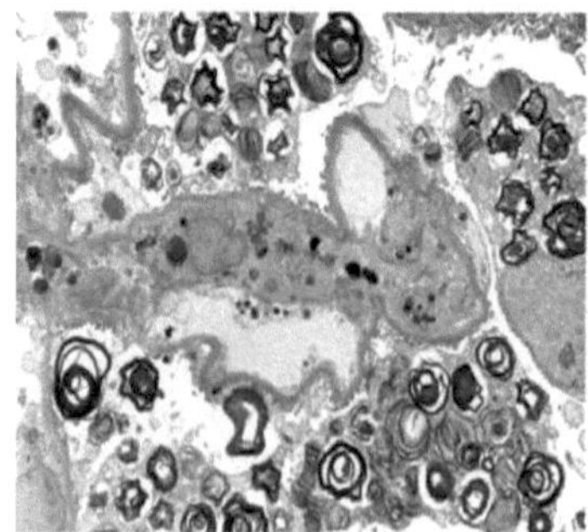

Figure 3: Tubular overload lesions. [22]

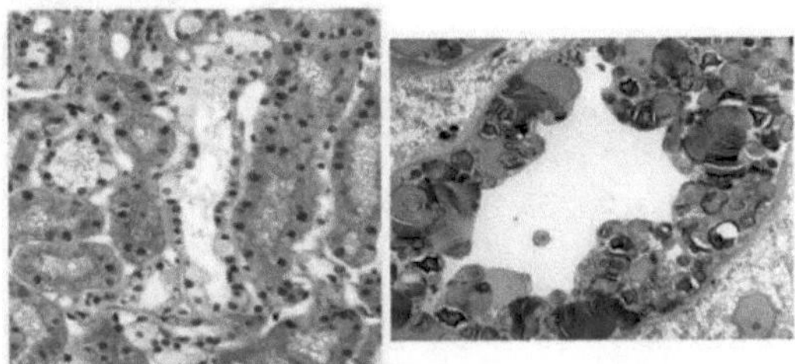

Figure 4: Tubular overload lesions in Fabry disease . [23]

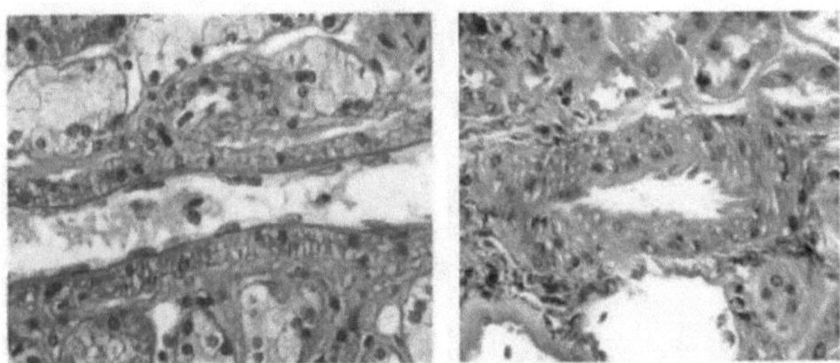

Figure 5: Arterial overload lesions in Fabry disease. [24]

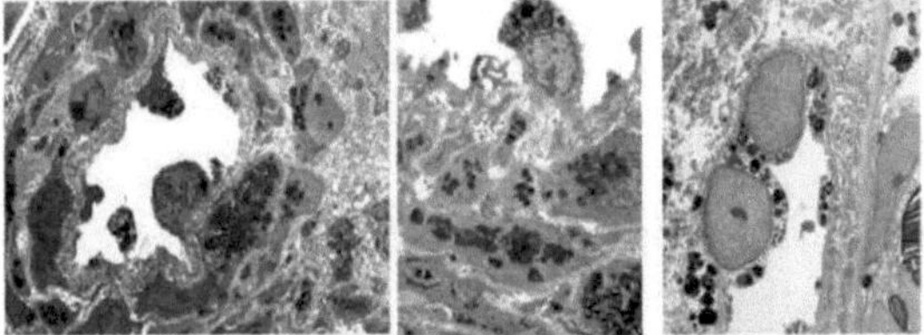

Figure: Arterial and capillary overload lesions in Fabry disease.[25]

b- In heterozygous women

Overload lesions in female subjects: Irregular involvement of the

- glomerular cells
- vascular and interstitial cells
- certain cells in the distal tubules

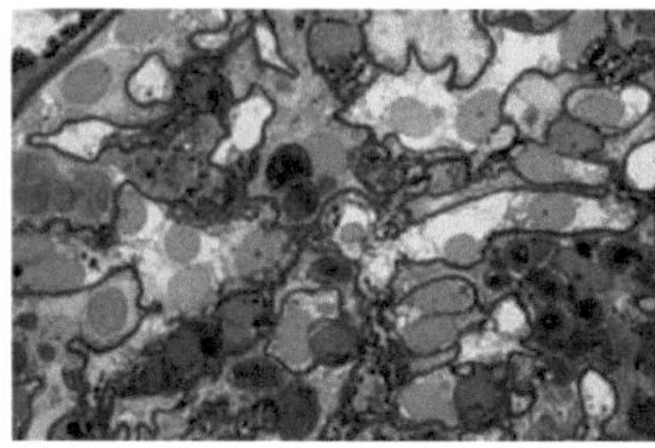

Figure 7: Irregular involvement in Fabry disease. [26]

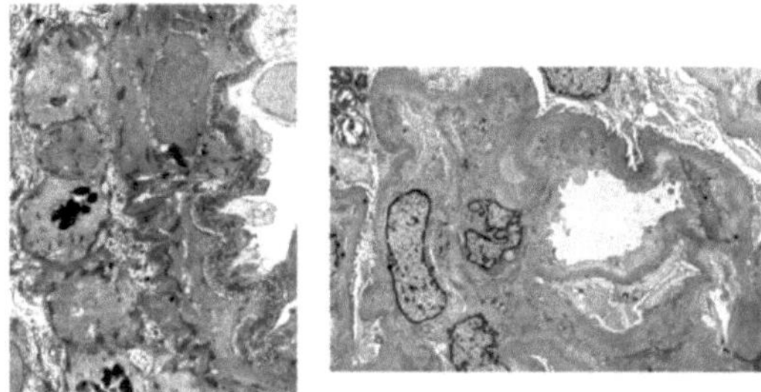

Figure 8 :Irregular cell overload in Fabry disease. [27]

Degenerative lesions :

– Myocyte necrosis > hyaline deposits and arteriolosclerosis

– Mesangial cell necrosis and segmental glomerulosclerosis

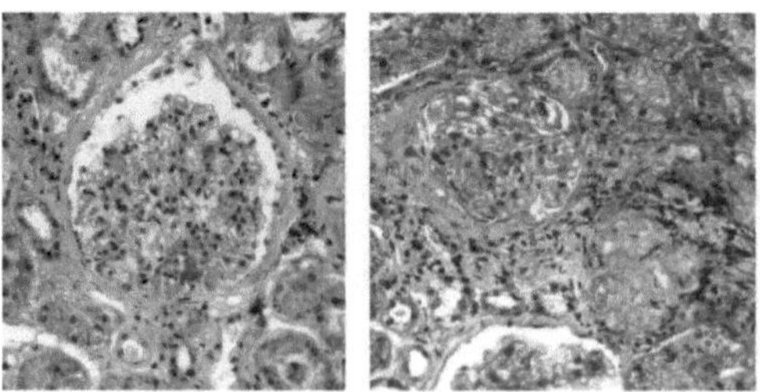

Figure 9: Progressive glomerulosclerosis in Fabry disease. [28]

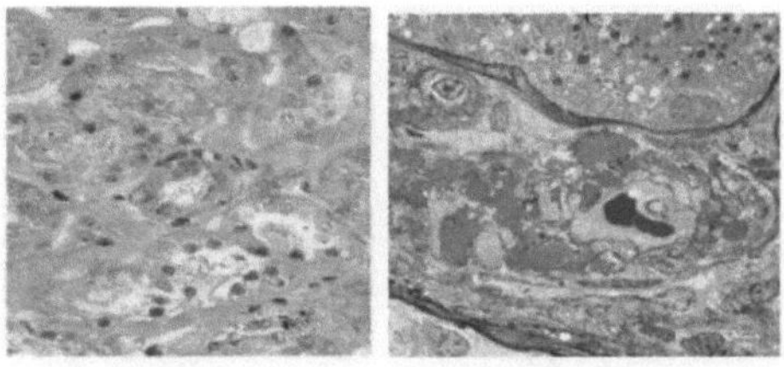

Figure 10: Necrosis of arterial myocytes in Fabry disease [29].

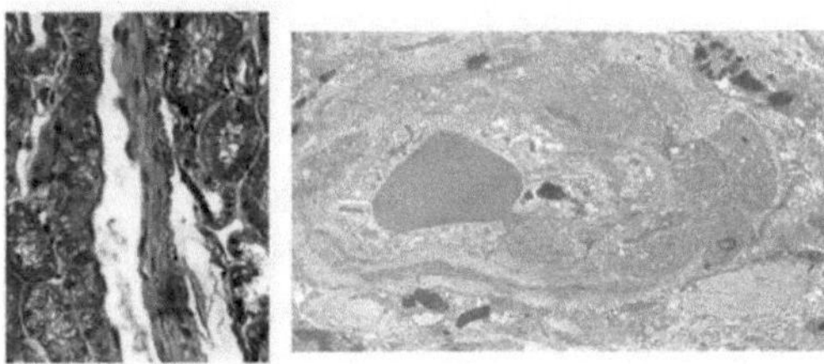

Figure11 :of arterial myocytes in Fabry disease . Figure [30]

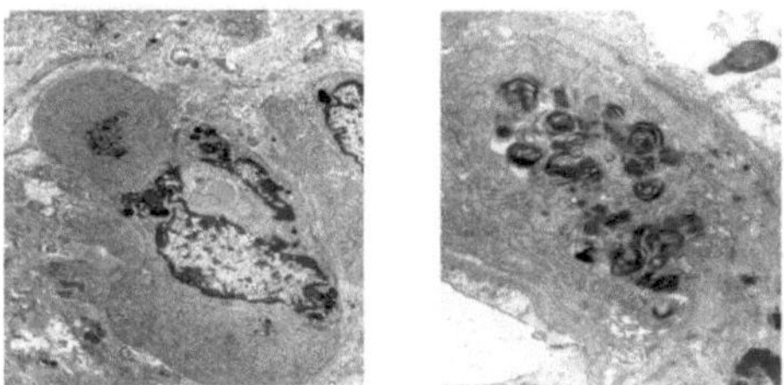

Figure 12: Arterial myocyte necrosis in Fabry disease . Figure [31]

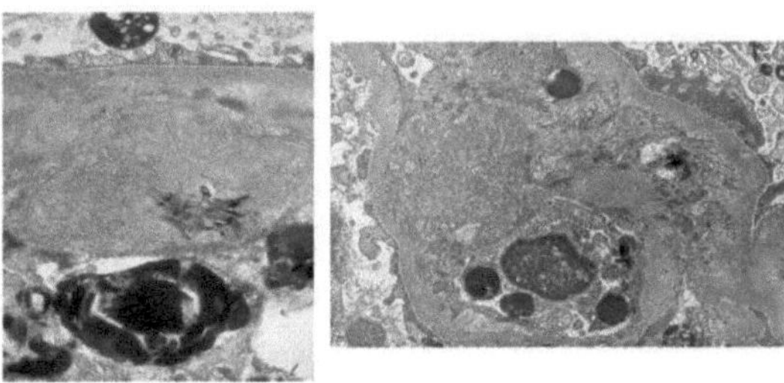

Figure 13: Mesangial cell necrosis in Fabry disease [32].

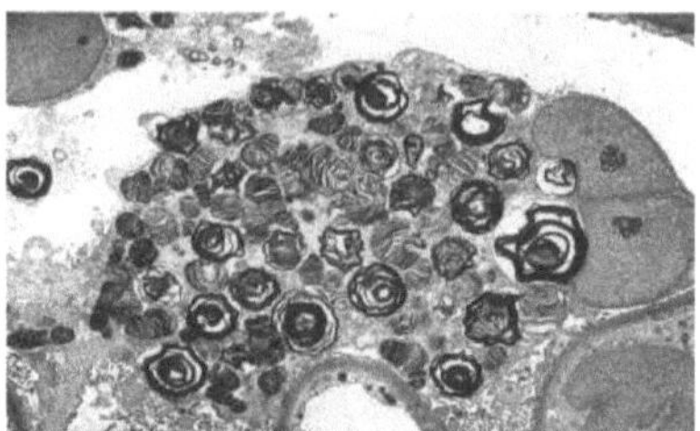

Figure14:Progressive progressive of the podocyte overload, podocyte alteration. Figure [33].

4- Treatment: enzyme replacement therapy enzyme replacement therapy is the current basis of treatment. It allows the decrease of inclusions of cells Alpha-galactosidase A [34] is given as a two-hour intravenous infusion at a dose of 0.2 mg/kg every 14 days.

5- a-galactosidase ß [35] is delivered by intravenous infusion over 2 to 4 hours, at a dose of 1mg/kg every 14 days.

- Effectiveness judged on

– clinical signs,

– renal function

– cardiac function,

– overload in endothelial cells

– plasma levels of globotriaosylceramide

B- Gaucher disease

1-Definition: This is an autosomal recessive disease linked to a deficit in an acidbetaglucosidase enzyme following a lysosomal accumulation of glucosylceramide in the cells of the reticuloendothelial system of the bone marrow, liver and spleen. Normally, glucocerebrosidase hydrolyses glucocerebrosides into glucose and ceramide. Genetic modifications to the enzyme lead t o accumulation of glucocerebroside in tissue macrophages through phagocytosis, forming Gaucher cells. The accumulation of Gaucher cells in the perivascular spaces of the brain leads to gliosis in the neurological form [36].

2-Clinical: the diagnosis is made on a myelogram or bone marrow biopsy, revealing Gaucher cells. It is confirmed by measuring leukocyte beta-glucocerebrosidase. Recently, a new marker has been identified, CCL18, a chemokine which is increased in this disease and correlated with renal impairment. Different types have been identified on the basis of the severity of clinical involvement. In the most common form (type 1), there is no mental or neurological impairment. All are linked to mutations in the same gene located on the chromosome 1. Usually, there is no clinical renal involvement apart from: Proteinuria in a few patients, in adulthood, after splenectomy or the presence of "Gaucher cells" in the flocculus, sometimes in the liver. intersitium, tubes and tubular lights. There are 3 types of Gaucher disease, which vary in terms of epidemiology, enzyme activity and manifestations.

Type I Gaucher disease: Type I (non-neuropathic) is very common (90% of all patients). Residual enzyme activity is highest. Ashkenazi Jews have the highest risk; 1/12 are carriers. Onset ranges from childhood to adulthood. Symptoms of type I Gaucher disease include hepatosplenomegaly, bone involvement (e.g. osteopenia, painful seizures, osteolytic lesions with fractures), growth retardation, delayed puberty, ecchymosis and pinguecula. Epistaxis and ecchymosis resulting from thrombocytopenia are common. X-rays showed twisting of the ends of the long bones (Erlenmeyer deformity) and cortical thinning[37].

Gaucher disease type II

Type II (acute neuropathic) is rare, and residual enzyme activity in this type is the lowest. Onset occurs in early childhood. The symptomatology of type II Gaucher disease is progressive neurological deterioration (e.g. rigidity, convulsions) with death by 2 years of age [38].

Type III Gaucher disease

Type III (subacute neuropathic) lies between types I and II in terms of incidence, enzyme activity and clinical severity. Onset occurs at any time during childhood. Clinical manifestations vary according to subtype and include progressive dementia and ataxia (IIIa), bone and visceral involvement (IIIb), and supranuclear palsies with corneal opacities (IIIc). Patients who survive into adolescence can live from many years [39].

3-Histology :

Voluminous Gaucher cells, cells with pale, finely granular cytoplasm, are visible in the subendothelial space and the stems of the glomerulus and in the interstitium.

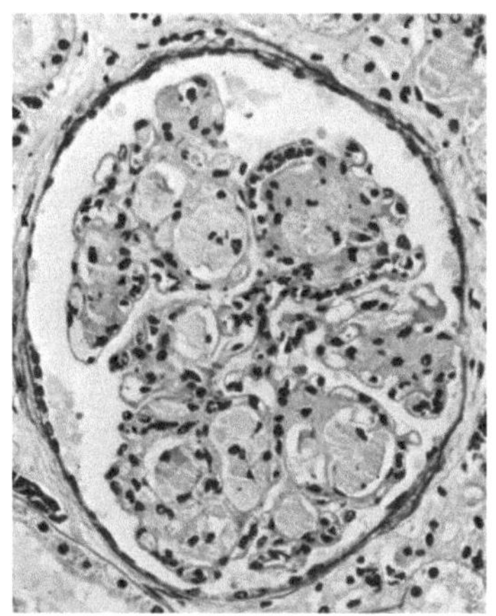

Figure 15: glomerular lesion in Gaucher's disease [40].

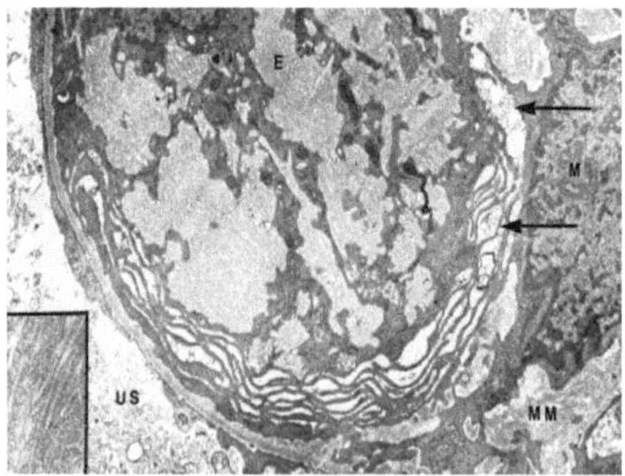

Figure 16: voluminous left-handed cells in ME [41].

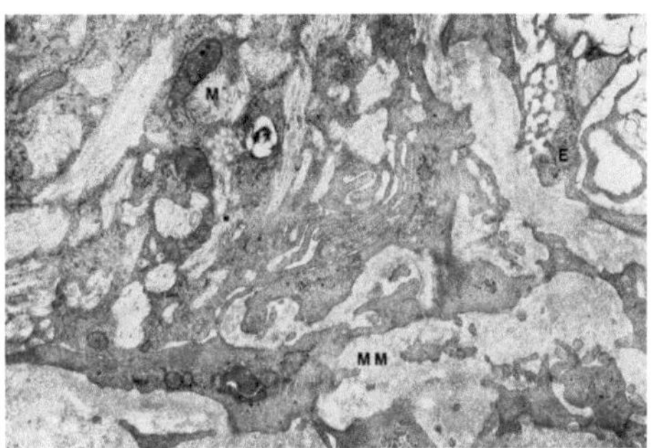

Figure 17: Left-handed lesion in ME [41].

C-Galactosialidosis

1-Definition:

This is another rare lysosomal storage disease. It is transmitted autosomal recessively.

2-Clinic

There are several clinical phenotypes which are classified as sialidosis type 1 non-dysmorphic, type II dysmorphic sialidosis with early onset in childhood or in utero. In severe type II forms with congenital or early infantile involvement . There is an oedematous syndrome, hepatosplenomegaly, sometimes with foetoplacental hydrops, neurological damage, facial dysmorphia, late skeletal anomalies, mental deterioration, ocular anomalies, cherry red spots, leading to early blindness. Renal failure may be associated with In the late infantile form, minor mental deterioration is sometimes present [42] . Biological diagnosis is based on the demonstration of a characteristic urinary oligosaccharide profile, which can be confirmed by measuring the activity of a-D-neura-minidase and other enzymes in fibroblasts or in utero. renal involvement in this thesaurisomosis is manifested by the early onset of proteinuria, followed by a nephrotic syndrome progressing over several years to end-stage renal failure [43] .

3- Histological lesions :

In type II sialidosis, podocytes and proximal tubular cells undergo massive and diffuse vacuolation. This has led to the identification of a new entity [44].

4- Treatment

In severe forms of type II sialidosis bone marrow and kidney transplantation may be proposed[45] .

2-Familial lecithin-cholesterol acyltransferase deficiency:

1-Definition :

Familial lecithin-cholesterol acyltransferase deficiency is a rare, autosomal recessive disease, initially described in Scandinavia where it is thought to be less exceptional - around 30 families have been described [46] . This enzyme, synthesised by the liver and then released into the plasma, is mainly associated with high-density lipoproteins (HDL) and those containing apolipoprotein B (very low-density lipoproteins or VLDL and low-density lipoproteins or LDL). Its deficiency leads to a defect in cholesterol esterification responsible for an accumulation of cholesterol in the tissue [47] . LCAT deficiency leads to abnormalities in the structure and composition of lipids and lipoproteins, in particular a significant increase in low-density lipoprotein (LDL) levels, which is probably responsible for the endothelial abnormalities observed. Mutations in the LCAT gene have been identified. Heterozygous cases are generally asymptomatic [48].

2 - The clinic

There are two forms of complete LCAT deficiency (Familial deficiency) in which there is a defect in the esterification of HDL and LDL and a partial deficiency.

a- Complete LCAT deficiency (Familial deficiency)

It is characterised by a number of symptoms: Corneal opacities in childhood, pseudo-gerotoxicity; normochromic anaemia in the 2nd decade linked to silent haemolysis, early atherosclerosis, hypertriglyceridaemia and calcifications in the 4th decade, and renal involvement, which is decisive for the prognosis of the disease and is revealed in childhood by proteinuria, sometimes associated with microscopic haematuria, which can be detected in childhood. Progression to renal failure is seen in the 4th and 5th decades. There is considerable phenotypic heterogeneity and recurrence may be seen in the transplanted kidney [49].

b- a defect in the esterification of HDL and LDL and a partial deficiency also known as **fish eye syndrome**, only the activity on HDL is altered [50].

3 - Genetic transmission :

The disease is transmitted in an autosomal recessive fashion, but sporadic cases have also been reported. Around forty mutations in the LCAT gene located on chromosome 16 at position q22.1 have been described, responsible for a partial or total deficiency of this enzyme. **Fish eye** disease may be linked to mutations in genes coding for apolipoprotein A [51].

4 histological studies

-Optical Microscopy :

It shows lesions secondary to the accumulation of lipids in the glomerulus. They are characterised by the presence of numerous and voluminous foam cells in the mesangium and endothelial cells with major vacuolisation. These vacuoles are empty. They can be better characterised on sections from frozen samples and are stained with oil red, a specific lipid stain. The walls are thickened segmentally by the lipid material, taking on a bullous appearance associated with enlargement of the mesangium, without proliferation of the cells. Segmental and focal hyalinosis lesions can be seen, as well as sub-endothelial deposits. Progression is towards global sclerosis. Foamy cells are seen in the interstitium. They have also been described in other organs such as the marrow and spleen. Arterioles often contain subendothelial deposits [52] .

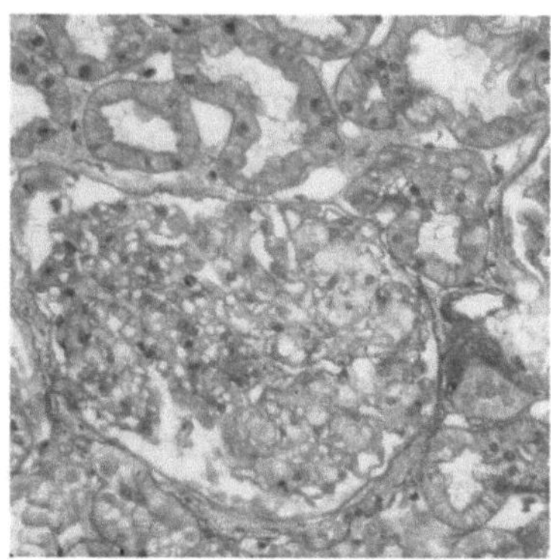

Figure 18: Familial lecithin-cholesterol acyltransferase deficiency lesions in MO [53].

It shows lesions secondary to the accumulation of lipids in the glomeruli. They are characterised by the presence of numerous, voluminous foam cells in the mesangium and endothelial cells with major vacuolisation. These vacuoles are empty. The specific stain is oil red, a specific lipid stain. The walls are thickened by lipid material in a segmental fashion, taking on a bullous appearance associated with enlargement of the mesangium, without cell proliferation. Segmental and focal hyalinosis lesions can be seen, as well as sub-endothelial deposits. Progression is towards global sclerosis [54].

-Immunofluorescence: negative. Arteriolar deposits of C3 can be seen.

-Electron microscopy: this reveals the cellular and extracellular accumulation of lipid deposits. In cells, they appear as small, dense osmiophilic membrane inclusions, distributed in large, partially empty vacuoles. In the extracellular matrix of the glomerulus, which they thicken, they are heterogeneous, consisting of an irregular association of dense membrane structures, amorphous flaky deposits and clear deposits. they are mainly observed in the capillary walls in a subendothelial position, pushing back the endothelial cells, and in the mesangial matrix. When the deposits are located in the thickness of the basal membrane or on the epithelial side, the dense component predominates. Lipid deposits of the same type are present under the endothelium of capillaries, arteries and veins [55]. Electron microscopy is not necessary to make a diagnosis. diagnosis.

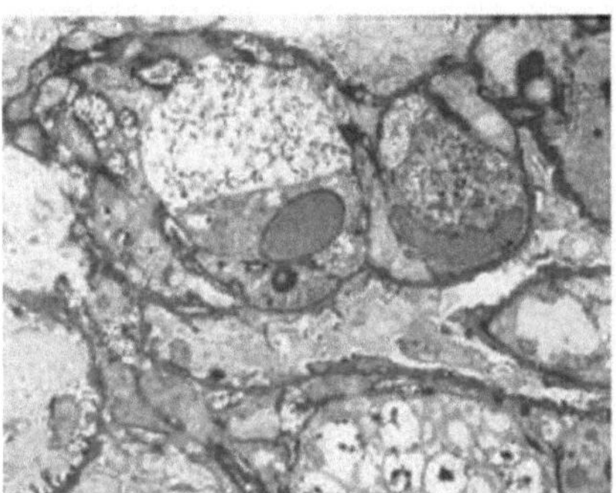

Figure 19: Complete LCAT deficiency by electron microscopy [56]:

Accumulation of lipid deposits in the cells: dense membrane inclusions within large "empty" vacuoles in the ECM of the glomerulus.

5- Differential diagnosis :

Superimposable renal lesions may be observed during familial hyperlipidaemia or in severe forms of Alagille syndrome. Light microscopy reveals vacuoles mainly in the mesangial stalks and in some subendothelial spaces. Electron microscopy reveals heterogeneous inclusions in the mesangial cells. Clear material containing osmiophilic membrane formations accumulates in the subendothelial space and in the glomerular mesangial rods. The lamina densa is preserved, but a few inclusions can be seen on the outer side of the glomerular wall [57].

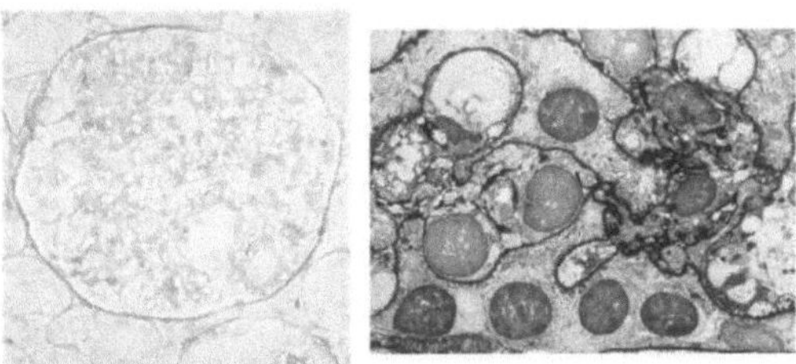

Figure 20: Differential diagnosis with lesions **of complete LCAT deficiency** [58] .

NB: similar lesions may be observed in various situations which share elevated serum levels of non-esterified cholesterol and phospholipids, and changes in lipoproteins: Alagille syndrome, severe HI, familial hypercholestorolaemia, type III hyperlipoproteinaemia (homozygotes for the E2 isoform of apoE).

6- Treatment

-Symptomatic treatment is recommended for affected patients. However, cases of recurrence have been reported, confirming the hypothesis that plasma lipid abnormalities are responsible for the lesions.

3-Lipoprotein glomerulopathy = glomerulopathy with lipoprotein deposits

This is a rare disease, described in Japan (Saito, 1989), which is characterised by a nephrotic syndrome without haematuria.Progression to ESRD is seen in half of patients.There are usually no extrarenal signs of lipid overload. There is a moderate increase in LDL and apo E The genetic mutation concerns ApoE mutations, most often located in the LDL receptor [59].

Clinical :

This nephropathy is due to an abnormality in the metabolism of apolipoproteine E (ApoE). A distinction is made between primary forms, which are inherited autosomal recessive, and secondary forms. In the primary forms, different types of ApoE mutation have been identified. Diagnosis is most often made in adulthood, and the disease is revealed by proteinuria, sometimes nephrotic. In 30/100 of cases, renal failure develops progressively. No abnormalities in lipid metabolism are found. There is sometimes an increase in B-lipoproteins and ApoE, without any extra-renal manifestations [60].

Histological study :

Light microscopy: distension and obstruction of glomerular capillaries by lipoprotein "thrombi", sometimes associated with voluminous mesangial deposits. They are weakly stained by PAS and very strongly stained by red oil. Foamy cells and vascular lesions are rare [61].

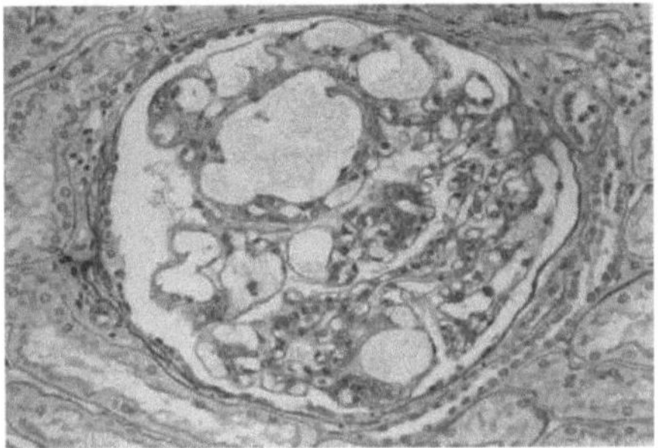

Figure 21: **Optical microscopy**: distension and obstruction of the glomerular capillaries by lipoprotein "thrombi" . [62]

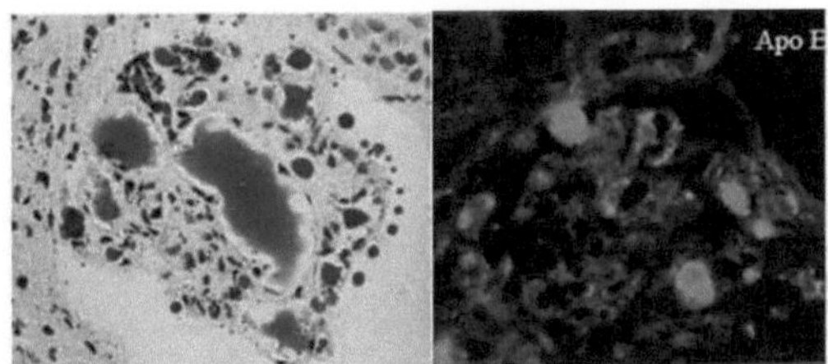

Figure 22: Lipoprotein glomerulopathy in IFI [63].

Immunofluorescence: the standard study is negative or non-specific with IGM and C3 deposits in the mesanguim, but it is possible to carry out immunostaining for B-lipoproteins or ApoE to confirm the nature of the deposits.

Electron microscopy: This visualises voluminous deposits consisting of innumerable granules of varying size and density, organised in states and giving a fingerprint-like image. Massive homogeneous mesangial deposits that are dense to electrons are associated with trhombi [64].

Treatment :

Cases of recurrence of the disease have been described after renal transplantation.

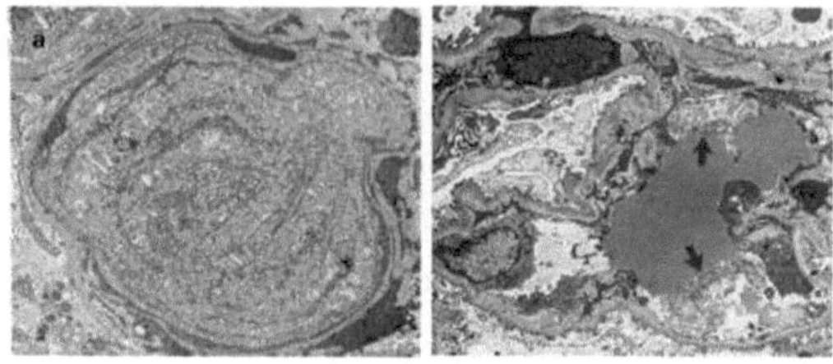

Figure 23: Lipoprotein glomerulopathy in ME. [65]

IV- TUBULOINTERSTITIAL NEPHROPATHY AND DISEASES "HEREDITARY' METABOLIC DISORDERS, OVERLOAD DISEASES

CLINICAL CASE 2 :

This was a 3-year-old child who presented in an emergency with convulsions in a febrile state following a recurrent urinary tract infection associated with vomiting and dehydration.

At the labstix: haematuria: ++.

Renal ultrasound: nephrocalcinosis Renal work-up: end-stage CKD.
ECG: heart rhythm disorder

AGT activity assay: collapsed AGXT gene mutation
Q1: What type of genetic disease

1-Cystinosis

Cystine is one of the fundamental constituents of proteins, and therefore of living matter. It is a small molecule that belongs to the amino acid family and contains sulphur[66].

Normally, cystine , which comes from the destruction of proteins, leaves the lysosome by crossing its wall. This is done with the help of a specific transporter, cystinosine , located in the wall of the lysosome .

It has recently been shown that it is the anomaly of this transporter which leads to the accumulation of cystine in the cell, the concentration of cystine being 50 to 100 times higher than normal. This accumulation can lead to crystallisation of cystine, which is 50 to 100 times higher than normal. This accumulation can lead toThe first organs affected are the kidney and the eye, followed by the thyroid gland, the pancreas, the liver, the spleen, the muscles and the nervous system[67].

Definition:

It is sufficiently rare to be classed as an orphan disease, but it is found in all countries. It has been known about since the beginning of the century, the first observation of a sick child being reported in 1903 by a German chemist, Abderhalden[68].

Later, observations of affected children made it possible to describe the various manifestations of the disease and to understand that cystinosis was :

- Characterised by insufficient reabsorption in the first portion of the tubule, the proximal convoluted tubule.
- Due to an accumulation of cystine in almost all cells

of the body.

- An inherited autosomal recessive disease. It was in 1955 that lysosomes, the structures present in all cells , were discovered.This discovery led to an understanding of the mechanisms of around fifty diseases known as lysosomal diseases, including cystinosis[69].

Different forms of cystinosis :

1 - **Infantile cystinosis**: represents the most frequent (1/100,000 - 1/200,000) and most severe form, accompanied by proximal tubulopathy. The age at which the first signs of renal involvement appear varies between 3 and 18 months. End-stage renal failure is constant in the absence of treatment. It used to occur before the age of 10, but early treatment with cysteamine considerably delays the onset of the disease [70].

Juvenile cystinosis: this is rarer, generally beginning in the second decade of life in children who had normal development up to that point, the onset of renal damage occurs late in life, and is characterised by glomerulopathy which progresses to end-stage renal failure [71].

Adult cystinosis: accompanied by isolated ocular involvement The three forms of the disease are allelic

The gene :

The gene was located in 1995 by the Cystinosis Collaborative Research Group in 17p- It was identified by C Antignac's team in 1998. This CTNS gene, with 12 exons, codes for a protein called [72].

Cystinosine

1- **infantile cystinosis**

Clinical symptoms of infantile cystinosis :

It is a proximal tubulopathy which appears between 3 and 6 months of age, and represents the most frequent cause of Fanconi syndrome in children. Progression to ESRD can be seen around the age of 8. It is associated with major growth retardation and ocular damage due to corneal deposits by the age of one year (1 year) and photophobia with retinal lesions and blindness by the age of 15-20 years [73].
Secondly, in children undergoing dialysis-transplantation, there are other disorders:

- Pancreatic disease and diabetes
- Thyroid disease and hypothyroidism
- Hepatomegaly and portal hypertension
- Delayed puberty and hypogonadism in boys
- Muscle and brain damage.

Biochemical diagnosis :

the biochemical **assay** measures the quantity of cystine accumulated inside the leucocyte, the cell in which cystine accumulates most strongly.

Clinical :

Tubular damage :

The renal tubule is the first to be affected. Cystinosis is an example.
Typical initial kidney lesions are :

- Irregularity of the epithelium of the proximal tubule without evidence of cystine crystals
- Podocytes are giant and multinucleated
- there is intralysosomal accumulation of cystine crystals with the presence of "dark cells" in electron microscopy [74].

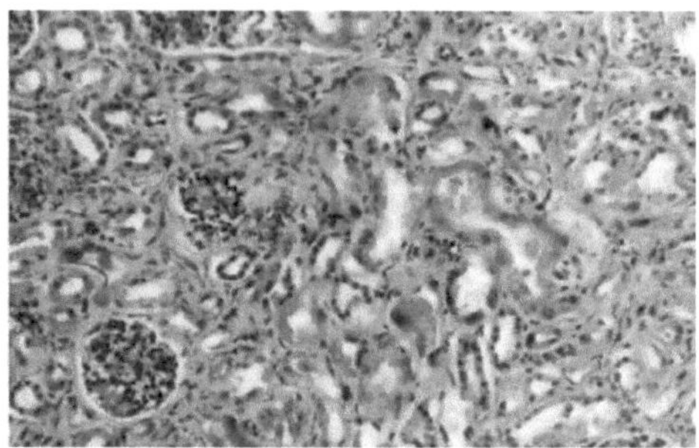

Figure 24: Irregularity of the proximal tubule epithelium without cystine crystals [75].

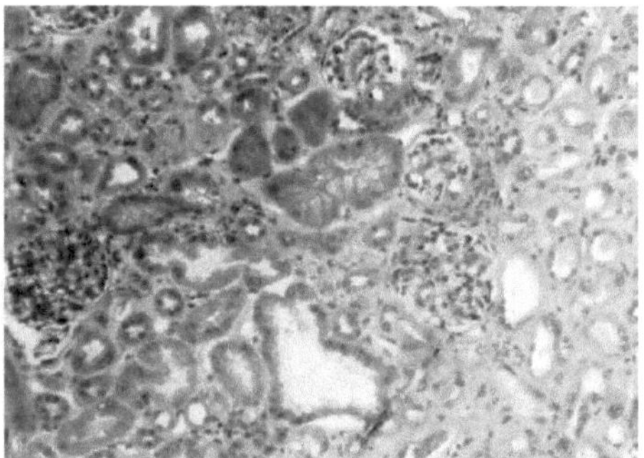

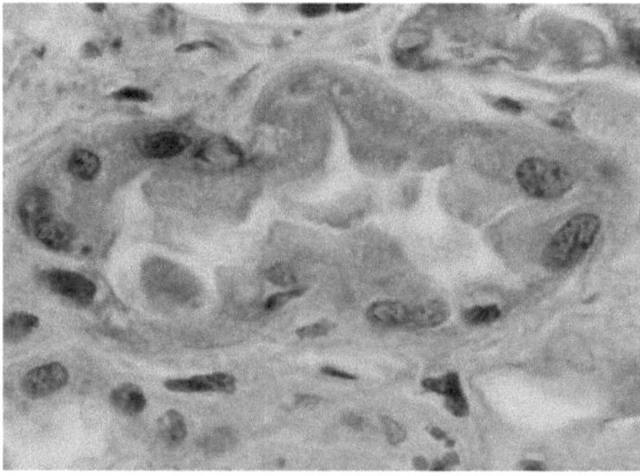

Figure 25Irregularity of the epithelium of the proximal tube in the absence of evidence of cystine crystals [76].

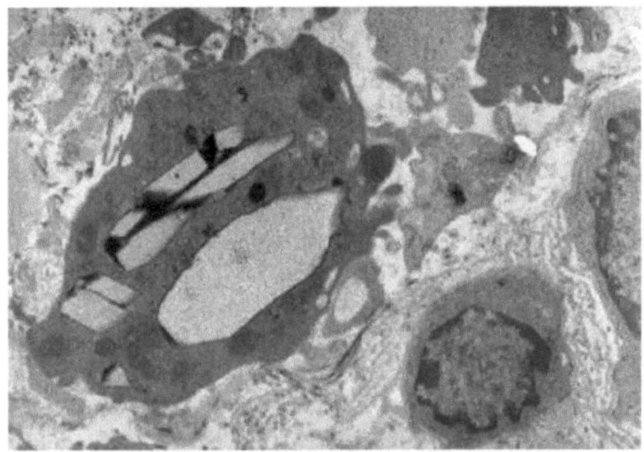

Figure 26 there is an intralysosomal accumulation of cystine crystals with the presence of "dark cells" in electron microscopy [77].

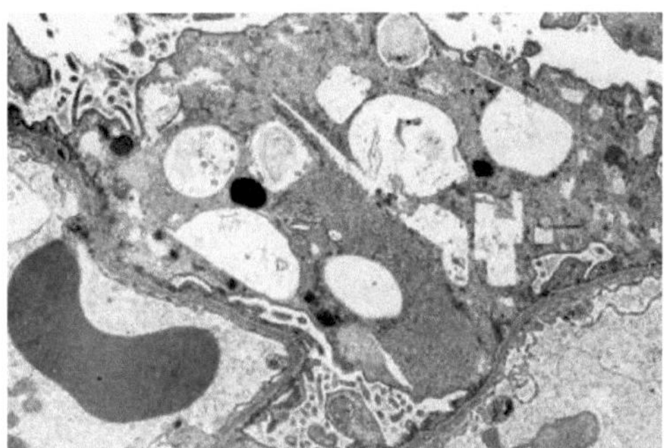

Figure 27 there is an intralysosomal accumulation of cystine crystals with the presence of "dark cells" in electron microscopy [78].

Secondary renal lesions are :

- Thickening of the arteriolar walls
- Hyperplasia of the juxtaglomerular apparatus
- Tubular atrophy, interstitial fibrosis
- Progressive glomerular alterations.

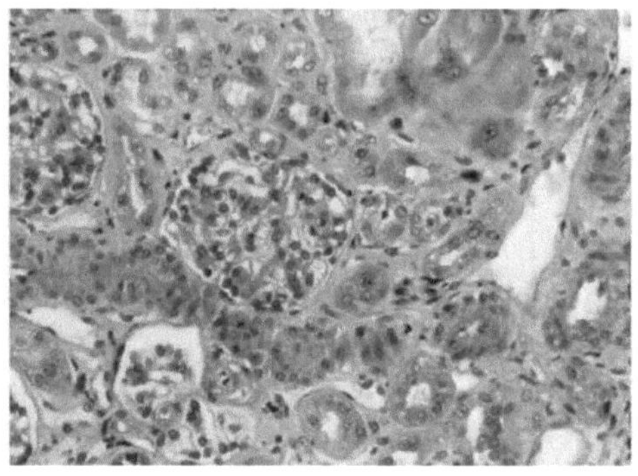

Figure28:secondary secondary at MO in cystinosis . [79]

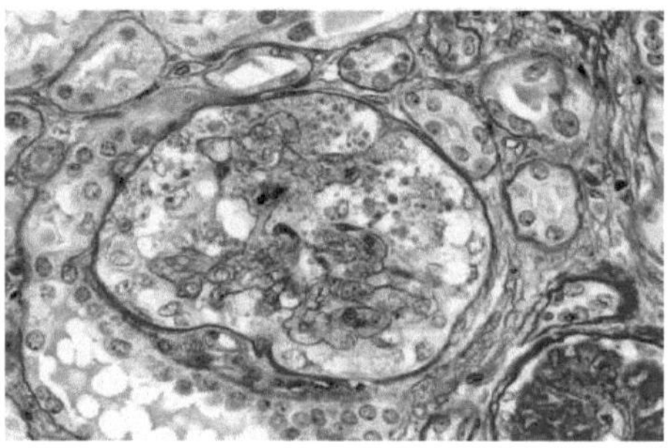

Figure29 : lesions secondary in MO in the cystinosis. [80]

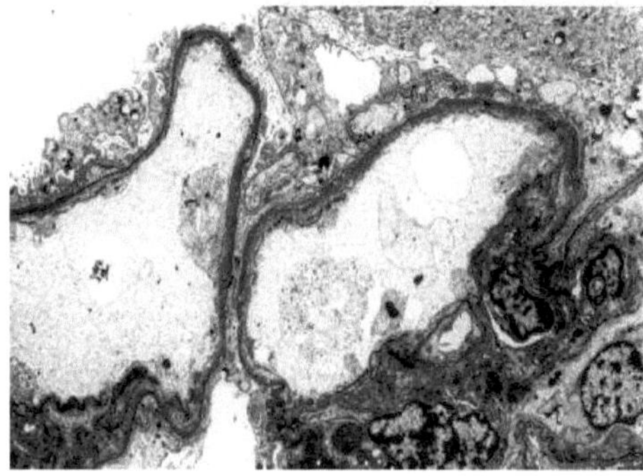

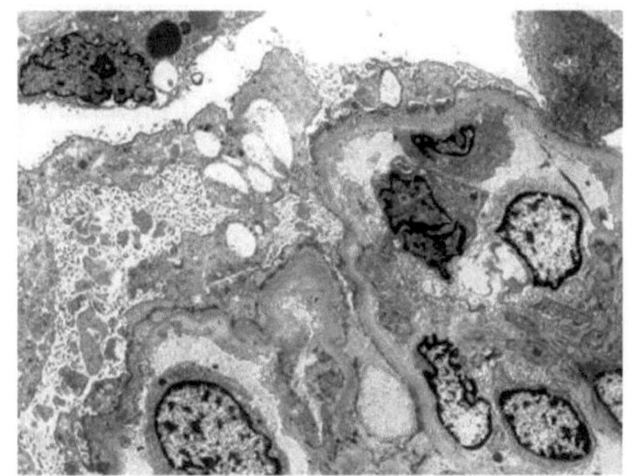

Figure30 : lesions secondary in ME in the cystinosis. [81]

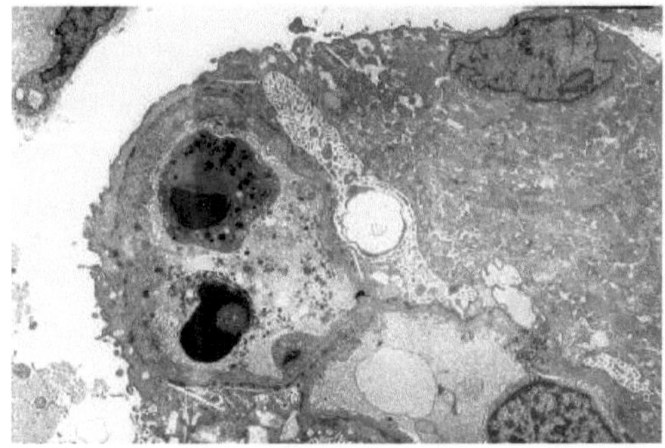

Figure 31: Secondary lesion in ME in cystinosis**[82]**

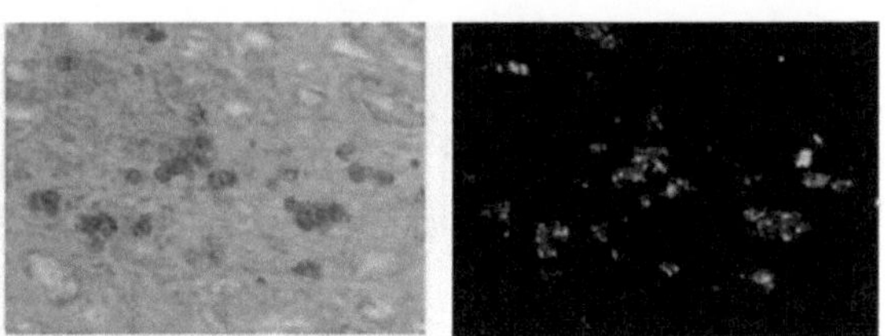

Figure 32: Accumulation of cystine crystals in the interstitium [83].

End kidney

Major cortico-medullary atrophy Massive renin synthesis

Transplanted kidney

There is no recurrence of symptoms or lesions after transplantation. Deposits of cystine crystals are sometimes found in the cells of the host infiltrating the graft, in the interstitium and mesangium with the presence of "black cells".

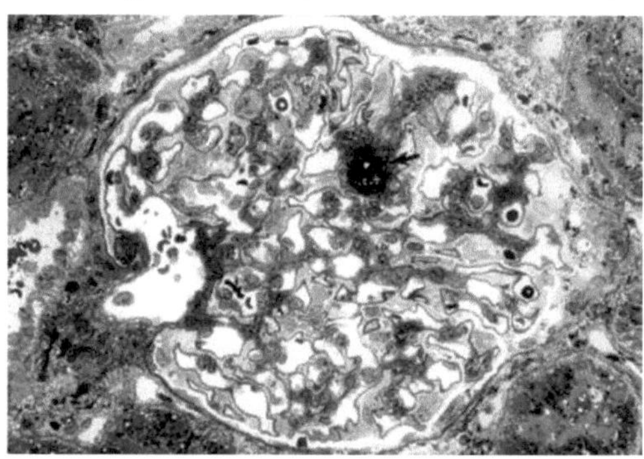

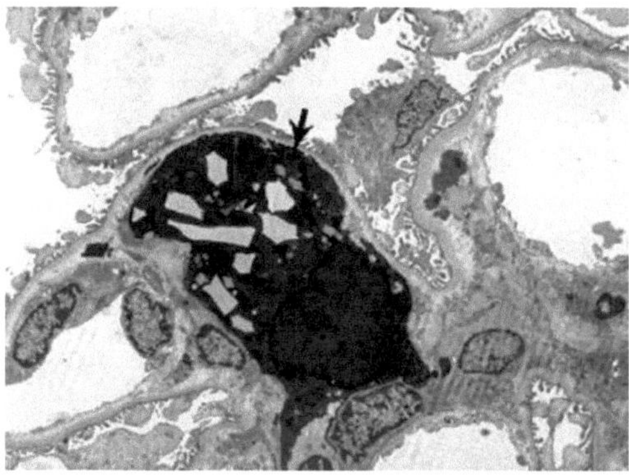

Figure 33: Presence of "black cells" in cystinosis .[84]

Treatment of infantile cystinosis

1 Symptomatic treatment: Symptomatic treatment is based on the different types of damage

-background treatment

Cysteamine (or its derivatives), which is administered very early on and on a regular and continuous basis, can delay the progression to ESRD. Its effect is only partially effective on tubulopathy, but it can prevent the systemic accumulation of cystine crystals.In mice, the results of stem cell transplantation are very promising [85].

II Juvenile cystinosis Clinical symptoms

Onset is delayed and occurs around the age of 12-15 years, usually characterised by glomerular proteinuria and absence or discretion of proximal tubular signs.

• progression to IRT occurs between the ages of 20 and 30 and is associated with corneal damage [86].

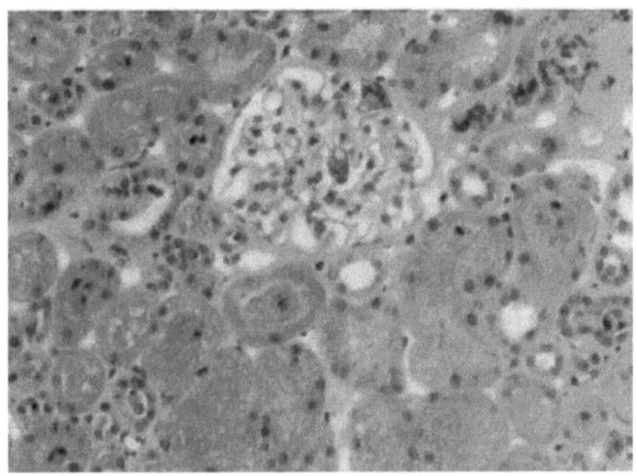

Figure 34: biopsy of juvenile cystinosis [87].

Cystinosine

Is a lysosomal protein characterised by the presence of two address signals to the lysosome, there are 7 potential glycosylation sites in the N-terminal part of the protein. The family of transporters with 7 transmembrane domains that transports cystine out of the lysosome. It is known as the cystine-proton symporter.

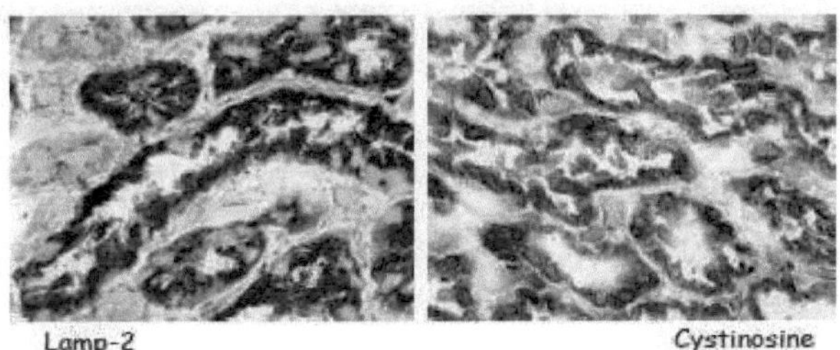

Figure35: Colocalization in proximal T cells of Lamp-2, a lysosomal marker, and cystinosin [88].

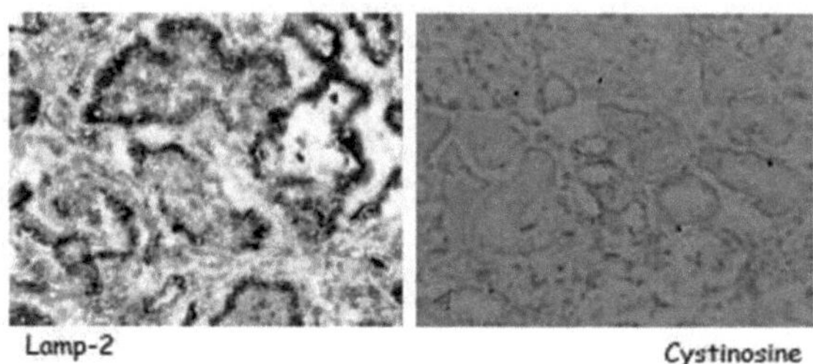

Figure 36: Absence of cystinosin in a patient with cystinosis. Normal expression of Lamp-2 [89] Conclusions

Proximal tubular lesions are the first renal lesions observed in patients with infantile cystinosis. The most striking feature is the virtual absence of crystals in the proximal tubular cells. Glomerular lesions become significant with the progression of the disease through specific podocyte damage or as a consequence of nephron reduction? Severe renal atrophy is observed in the end stage. It is characterised by the intensity of arterial and arteriolar lesions associated with significant renin synthesis (explaining the frequent hypertension at this stage). There is an accumulation of cystine crystals in the interstitial cells of the corticomedullary junction. There is no recurrence of specific tubular or glomerular lesions in the transplanted kidney.

Clinical case 3

The patient was a 3-year-old child who presented to the emergency department with convulsions in a febrile state following a recurrent urinary tract infection associated with vomiting and dehydration.
At the labstix: haematuria: ++.

Renal ultrasound: nephrocalcinosis Renal work-up: end-stage CKD. ECG: heart rhythm disorder AGT activity assay: collapsed AGXT gene mutation

Q1: What type of genetic disease?

2- **Primary oxalosis or hyperoxaluria**

There are three types of primary hyperoxaluria: type 1, which is themost frequentform (1/60,000-1/200,000 births) type 2, which is rare and mainly responsible for lithiasis type 3, which is exceptional and linked to hyper-absorption of oxalate. Can found des hyperoxaluria secondarya several mechanisms:By absorption of foods rich in oxalates following an intestinal resection or by metabolic dysfunction, or by changes in intestinal flora (prolonged antibiotic treatment or transplant patients).

Primary oxalosis or hyperoxaluria type 1 Definitions

This is an autosomal recessive disease characterised by a defect in a hepatic enzyme, the peroxisomal AGT or alanine glyoxylate aminotransferase, whose co-enzyme is vitamin B6. This is not a primarily renal disease, but the renal (and extra-renal) consequence of a hereditary metabolic disease linked to the excessive production of oxalic acid[90]. The preferential but not exclusive target of calcium oxalate crystalline deposits is the kidney, as poorly soluble oxalates are not metabolised but excreted in the urine, leading to the formation of lithiasis and the appearance of nephrocalcinosis.

Genetic study

The AGXT gene has 11 exons and is located at 2q37.3. Mutations in the gene most often lead to an absence of protein, inactivity or abnormal localisation (mitochondrial) of the mutated protein. Specific mutations have been observed in certain ethnic groups, indicating a founder effect [91].

Clinical presentation :

1 **The infantile form**: is a rare formcharacterised by nephrocalcinosis and early ESRD.

2 **Late form**: characterised by the appearance of a few stones. in adults and the elderly.

The usual form generally involves recurrent urinary lithiasis and progressive IR, leading to diagnosis in childhood or adolescence.

Histological study :

The renal biopsy shows intra-tubular and then diffuse deposits of calcium oxalate with progressive destruction of the renal parenchyma

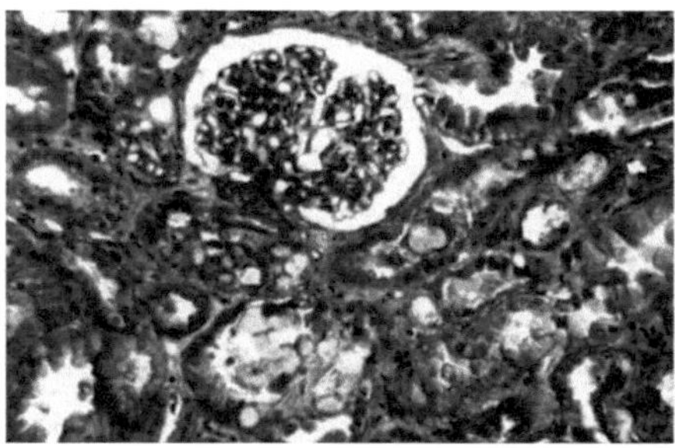

Figure 37: MO lesion of oxalosis

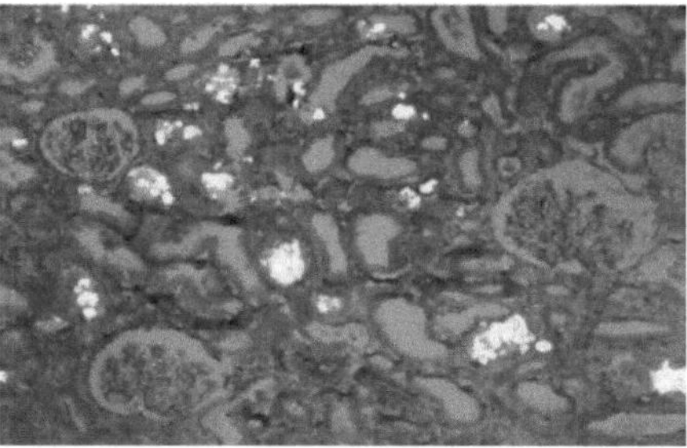

Figure 38: oxalosis lesion

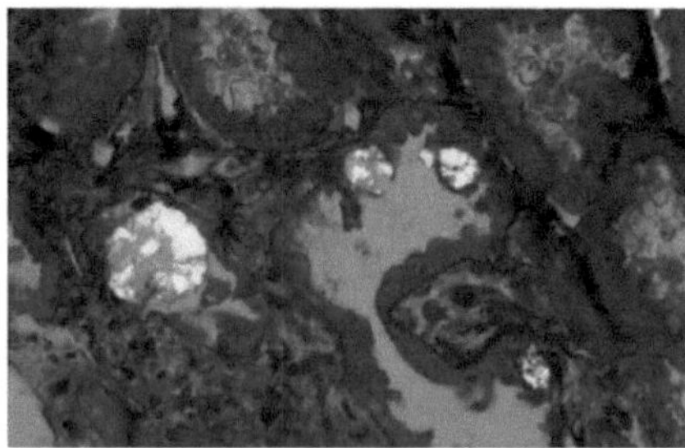

Figure 39: Calcium oxalate crystal lesion

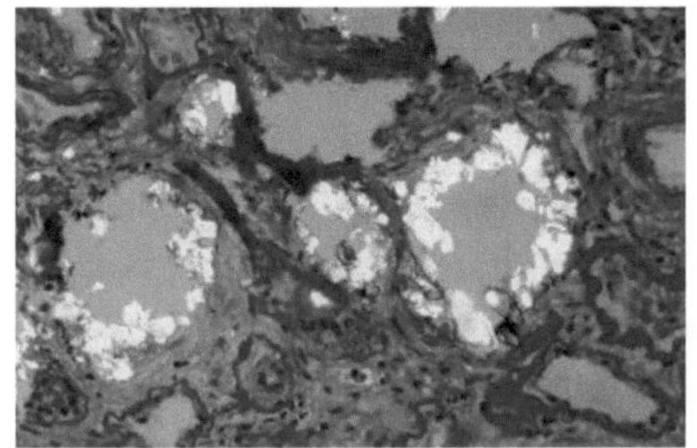

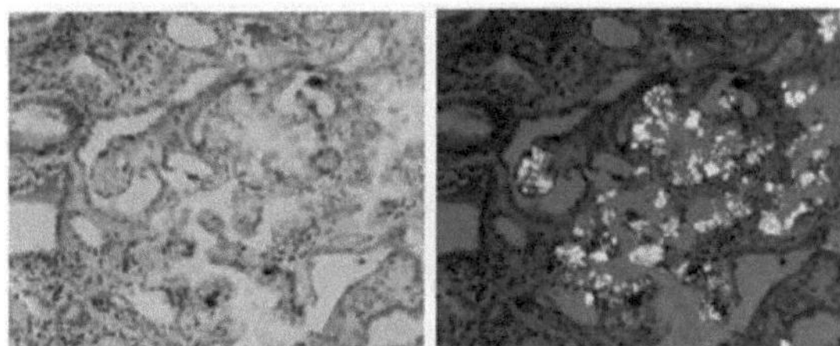

Figure 40: Calcium oxalate lesion

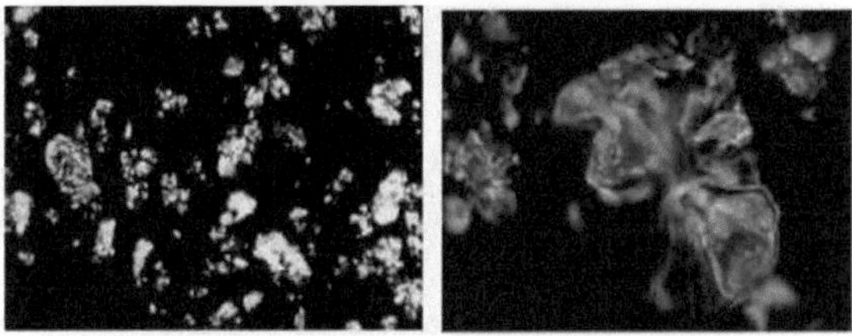

Figure 41 Calcium oxalate crystals

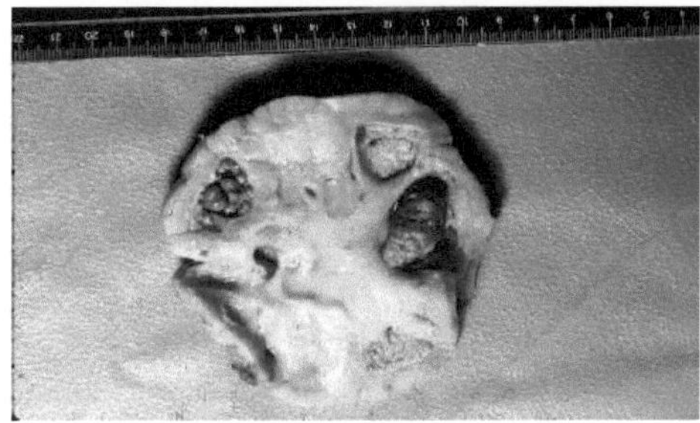

Extrarenal manifestations

When the glomerular filtration rate falls below 40-50mL/mn/1.73 m2 and the plasma oxalate concentration exceeds 30-50µmol/L, extra-renal symptoms appear: osteoarticular damage, cardiovascular damage with rhythm disorders and arterial calcifications, bilateral retinal eye damage and damage to the skin and mucous membranes Oxalate deposits are generally deposited in all tissues, making it a particularly painful and disabling disease [98].

Progression after renal transplantation

Recurrence in the transplanted kidney is constant, and occurs earlier and in greater numbers the longer the patient has been on haemodialysis.

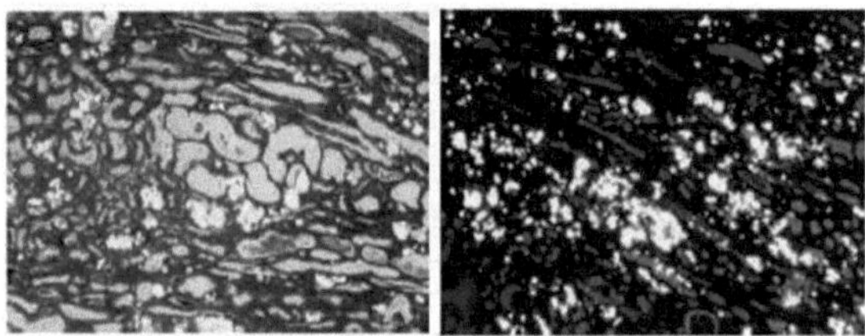

Oxalosis: recurrence in transplanted kidney

Liver transplantation before the stage of end-stage renal failure corrects the enzyme deficiency, while combined liver-kidney transplantation is rare; there are around 10 per year worldwide [100].

3- Glycogenoses :

Glycogenosis results from abnormalities in the enzymes involved in the degradation of glycogen, the macromolecule used to store glucose. Thesaurisomas are genetic diseases of carbohydrate metabolism leading to the accumulation of glycogen, mainly in the liver, muscles and sometimes the kidney. nine varieties have been identified. They are all autosomal recessive except for type VII which is X-linked [101].

Clinical :

It sometimes manifests itself as severe hypoglycaemia at birth, but can occur later, between three and four months of age, accompanied b y other biological abnormalities such as acidosis lactic acidosis, hyperlipidaemia and hyperuricaemia [102]. Affected children have a doll's face with thin limbs due to amyotrophy, delayed stature, hepatomegaly and severe fatigue due to early hypoglycaemia. Lipomas and diarrhoea are common, as well as macroglossia, respiratory infections and haemorrhagic manifestations due to thrombopathy. In the absence of treatment, the disease progresses with insufficient growth, bone demineralisation, delayed puberty, gout or lithiasis due to hyperuricaemia, pancreatic insufficiency, pulmonary arterial hypertension and renal manifestations [103].

Histological lesions :

Kidney biopsies are performed only in exceptional cases; glomeruli are increased in size and fibrous lesions with glomerulosclerosis may be present. Significant clarification of podocytes, proximal tubules and endothelial cells is observed. PAS staining confirms the accumulation of glycogen in these cell types, and the nuclei sometimes contain glycogenic inclusions. Electron microscopy reveals optically empty vacuoles in the cytoplasm of the cells [104].

Pathophysiology :

Glycogenes are the result of an accumulation of glycogen, whether normal or abnormal, within several organs. This is the result of congenital deficiency of one or more enzymes involved in glycogen metabolism [105] .

Treatment

It involves eating frequent meals rich in slow sugars and protein. Hypoglycaemia is treated symptomatically. In addition , Allopurinol may be proposed as soon as uricemia is high, as well as alkalinisation if the venous bicarbonate concentration is less than 20 ml/l, and the use of a conversion enzyme inhibitor to reduce microalbuminuria or proteinuria [106].

CONCLUSION

Genetic kidney diseases (GKDs) are rare diseases (with the exception of polycystic kidney disease) that are inherited. Individually, they represent only a small proportion of kidney diseases, but given the large number of diseases identified, the total number of patients suffering from them is high. GDMs include diseases that primarily affect the kidneys, but also those that affect the whole body, including the kidneys, and require follow-up by a nephrology specialist.

REFERENCES

1. Futerman AH, Van Meer G. The cell biology of lysosomal storage disease. Nat Rev Mol Cell Biol 2004; 5 : 554-65. [Google Scholar]

2. Raas-Rothschild A, Pankova-Kholmyansky I, Kacher Y, Futerman AH. Glycosphingolipidoses: beyond the enzymatic defect. Glycoconj J 2004; 21: 295-304.

3. Deegan PB, Baehner AF, Barba Romero MA, Hughes DA, Kampmann C, Beck M; European FOS Investigators. Natural history of Fabry disease in females in the Fabry Outcome Survey. J Med Genet. 2006 Apr;43(4):347-52. doi: 10.1136/jmg.2005.036327. Epub 2005 Oct 14. Citation on PubMed or Free article on PubMed Central

4. Desnick RJ, Brady R, Barranger J, Collins AJ, Germain DP, Goldman M, Grabowski G, Packman S, Wilcox WR. Fabry disease, an under-recognized multisystemic disorder: expert recommendations for diagnosis, management, and enzyme replacement therapy. Ann Intern Med. 2003 Feb 18;138(4):338-46. doi: 10.7326/0003-4819-138-4-200302180-00014. Citation on PubMed

5. Eng CM, Germain DP, Banikazemi M, Warnock DG, Wanner C, Hopkin RJ, Bultas J, Lee P, Sims K, Brodie SE, Pastores GM, Strotmann JM, Wilcox WR. Fabry disease: guidelines for the evaluation and management of multi-organ system involvement. Genet Med. 2006 Sep;8(9):539-48. doi: 10.1097/01.gim.0000237866.70357.c6. Citation on PubMed

6. Feldt-Rasmussen U, Rasmussen AK, Mersebach H, Rosenberg KM, Hasholt L, Sorensen SA. Fabry disease--a metabolic disorder with a challenge for endocrinologists? Horm Res. 2002;58(6):259-65. doi: 10.1159/000066443. Citation on PubMed

7. Hauser AC, Lorenz M, Sunder-Plassmann G. The expanding clinical spectrum of Anderson-Fabry disease: a challenge to diagnosis in the novel era of enzyme replacement therapy. J Intern Med. 2004 Jun;255(6):629-36. doi: 10.1111/j.1365-2796.2004.01300.x. Citation on PubMed

8. Mehta A, Hughes DA. Fabry Disease. 2002 Aug 5 [updated 2023 Mar 9]. In: Adam MP, Feldman J, Mirzaa GM, Pagon RA, Wallace SE, Bean LJH, Gripp KW, Amemiya A, editors. GeneReviews(R) [Internet]. Seattle (WA): University of Washington, Seattle; 1993-2023. Available from http://www.ncbi.nlm.nih.gov/books/NBK1292/

Citation on PubMed

9. Spada M, Pagliardini S, Yasuda M, Tukel T, Thiagarajan G, Sakuraba H, Ponzone A, Desnick RJ. High incidence of later-onset fabry disease revealed by newborn screening. Am J Hum Genet. 2006 Jul;79(1):31-40. doi: 10.1086/504601. Epub 2006 Apr 28. Citation on PubMed or Free article on PubMed Central

10. Wang RY, Lelis A, Mirocha J, Wilcox WR. Heterozygous Fabry women are not just carriers, but have a significant burden of disease and impaired quality of life. Genet Med. 2007 Jan;9(1):34-45. doi: 10.1097/gim.0b013e31802d8321. Citation on PubMed

11. M.H. Branton, R. Schiffmann, S.G. Sabnis, et al.

12. Natural history of Fabry renal disease: influence of alpha-galactosidase A activity and genetic mutation on clinical course.Medicine (Baltimore), 81 (2002), pp. 122

13. G. Houge, A.J. Skarbovik.Fabry disease a diagnostic and therapeutic challenge.Tidsskr Nor Laegefore, 125 (2005), pp. 1004

14. M. Spada, S. Pagliardini, M. Yasuda, et al.High incidence of later-onset fabry disease revealed by newborn screening.Am J Hum Genet, 79 (2006), pp. 31

15. W.L. Hwu, Y.H. Chien, N.C. Lee, et al.Newborn screening for Fabry disease in Taiwan reveals a high incidence of the later-onset GLA mutation c.936- 919.Hum Mutat, 30 (2009), pp

16. A. Mehta, M. Beck, F. Eyskens, et al.Fabry disease: a review of current management strategies.QJM, 103 (2010), pp. 641

17. S. Waldek, S. Feriozzi.Fabry nephropathy: a review-how can we optimize the management of Fabry nephropathy?BMC Nephrol, 15 (2014), pp. 72

18. Desnick RJ, Brady R, Barranger J et al. Fabry disease, an under-recognized multisystemic disorder: expert recommendations for diagnosis, management, and enzyme replacement therapy. Ann Intern Med 2003; 138: 338-346.

19. Thadhani R, Wolf M, West ML et al. Patients with Fabry disease on dialysis in the United States. Kidney Int 2002; 61: 249-255. 3. Meikle PJ, Hopwood JJ, Clague AE et al. Prevalence of lysosomal storage disorders. JAMA 1999; 281: 249-254.

20. Deegan PB, Baehner AF, Barba Romero MA et al. Natural history of Fabry disease in females in the Fabry Outcome Survey. J Med Genet 2006; 43: 347- 352.

21. Wang RY, Lelis A, Mirocha J et al. Heterozygous Fabry women are not just carriers, but have a significant burden of disease and impaired quality of life. Genet Med 2007; 9: 34-45.
22. Berg K. Inactivation of one of the X chromosomes in females is a biological phenomenon of clinical importance. Acta Med Scand 1979; 206: 1-3.
23. Dobrovolny R, Dvorakova L, Ledvinova J et al. Relationship between X-inactivation and clinical involvement in Fabry heterozygotes. Eleven novel mutations in the alpha-galactosidase A gene in the Czech and Slovak population. J Mol Med 2005; 83: 647-654.
24. Wilcox WR, Oliveira JP, Hopkin RJ et al. Females with Fabry disease frequently have major organ involvement: lessons from the Fabry Registry. Mol Genet Metab 2008; 93: 112-128.
25. Ortiz A, Oliveira JP, Waldek S et al. Nephropathy in males and females with Fabry disease: cross-sectional description of patients before treatment with enzyme replacement therapy. Nephrol Dial Transplant 2008; 23: 1600-1607
26. Desnik RJ, Ioannou YA, Eng MC. a-galactose A deficiency: Fabry disease. In: Scriver CR, Beaudet AL, Shy WS, Valle D, editors. The metabolic and molecular bases of Inherited diseases. 8th ed. McGraw Hill Book; 2001. pp. 3733-74. chapter 150 [Google Scholar].
27. Amin SS, Jahseen M, Ahamed Z, Zaheer MS, Perwin N. Angiokeratoma corporis diffusum (Fabry's disease) JIACM. 2004;5:79-82. [Google Scholar]
28. Rahman P, Gladman DD, Wither J, Silver MD. Coexistence of Fabry's disease and systemic lupus erythematosus. Clin Exp Rheumatol. 1998;16:475-
8. [PubMed] [Google Scholar]

29. Paira SO, Roverano S, Iribas JL, Barceló HA. Joint manifestations of Fabry's disease. Clin Rheumatol. 1992;11:562-5. [PubMed] [Google Scholar]
30. Martinez P, Aggio M, Rozenfeld P. High incidence of autoantibodies in Fabry disease patients. J Inherit Metab Dis. 2007;30:365-9. [PubMed] [Google Scholar]
31. Rosenmann E, Kobrin I, Cohen T. Kidney involvement in systemic lupus erythematosus and Fabry's disease. Nephron. 1983;34:180-.
4. [PubMed] [Google Scholar]

32. Arias Martínez N, Barbado Hernández FJ, Pérez Martí;n G, Pérez de Ayala C, Casal Esteban V, Vázquez Rodrí;guez JJ. Fabry's disease associated with

rheumatoid arthritis. Multisystemic crossroads. An Med Interna. 2003:20, 28-30. [PubMed] [Google Scholar]

33. Lacomis D, Roeske-Anderson L, Mathie L. Neuropathy and Fabry's disease. Muscle Nerve. 2005;31:102-7. [PubMed] [Google Scholar]
34. Schiffmann R. Neuropathy and Fabry disease: Pathogenesis and enzyme replacement therapy. Acta Neurol (Belq) 2006;160:61-5. [PubMed] [Google Scholar]
35. 12. Eng CM, Guffon N, Wilcox WR, Germain DP, Lee P, Waldek S, et al. Safety and efficacy of recombinant human alpha-galactosidase A replacement therapy in Fabrys disease. N Engl J Med. 2001;345:9-16. [PubMed] [Google Scholar]
36. Beutler E. Gaucher disease: multiple lessons from a single gene disorder. Acta Paediatr Suppl. 2006 Apr;95(451):103-9. doi: 10.1080/08035320600619039. Citation on PubMed
37. Chabas A, Cormand B, Grinberg D, Burguera JM, Balcells S, Merino JL, Mate I, Sobrino JA, Gonzalez-Duarte R, Vilageliu L. Unusual expression of Gaucher's disease: cardiovascular calcifications in three sibs homozygous for the D409H mutation. J Med Genet. 1995 Sep;32(9):740-2. doi: 10.1136/jmg.32.9.740. Citation on PubMed or Free article on PubMed Central
38. Eblan MJ, Goker-Alpan O, Sidransky E. Perinatal lethal Gaucher disease: a distinct phenotype along the neuronopathic continuum. Fetal Pediatr Pathol. 2005 Jul-Oct;24(4-5):205-22. doi: 10.1080/15227950500405296. Citation on PubMed

39. George R, McMahon J, Lytle B, Clark B, Lichtin A. Severe valvular and aortic arch calcification in a patient with Gaucher's disease homozygous for the D409H mutation. Clin Genet. 2001 May;59(5):360-3. doi: 10.1034/j.1399- 0004.2001.590511.x. Citation on PubMed
40. Grabowski GA, Andria G, Baldellou A, Campbell PE, Charrow J, Cohen IJ, Harris CM, Kaplan P, Mengel E, Pocovi M, Vellodi A. Pediatric non- neuronopathic Gaucher disease: presentation, diagnosis and assessment. Consensus statements. Eur J Pediatr. 2004 Feb;163(2):58-66. doi: 10.1007/s00431-003-1362-0. Epub 2003 Dec 16. Citation on PubMed

41. Kurolap A, Del Toro M, Spiegel R, Gutstein A, Shafir G, Cohen IJ, Barrabes JA, Feldman HB. Gaucher disease type 3c: New patients with unique presentations and review of the literature. Mol Genet Metab. 2019 Jun;127(2):138-146. doi: 10.1016/j.ymgme.2019.05.011. Epub 2019 May 21. Citation on PubMed

42. Groener J, Maaswinkel-Mooy P, Smit V, van der Hoeven M, Bakker J, Campos Y, d'Azzo A. New mutations in two Dutch patients with early infantile galactosialidosis. Mol Genet Metab. 2003 Mar;78(3):222-8. doi: 10.1016/s1096-7192(03)00005-2. Citation on PubMed
43. Malvagia S, Morrone A, Caciotti A, Bardelli T, d'Azzo A, Ancora G, Zammarchi E, Donati MA. New mutations in the PPBG gene lead to loss of PPCA protein which affects the level of the beta-galactosidase/neuraminidase complex and the EBP-receptor. Mol Genet Metab. 2004 May;82(1):48-55. doi: 10.1016/j.ymgme.2004.02.007. Citation on PubMed
44. Matsumoto N, Gondo K, Kukita J, Higaki K, Paragison RC, Nanba E. A case of galactosialidosis with a homozygous Q49R point mutation. Brain Dev. 2008 Oct;30(9):595-8. doi: 10.1016/j.braindev.2008.01.012. Epub 2008 Apr 18. Citation on PubMed

45. Nobeyama Y, Honda M, Niimura M. A case of galactosialidosis. Br J Dermatol. 2003 Aug;149(2):405-9. doi: 10.1046/j.1365-2133.2003.05488.x. Citation on PubMed

46. Funke H, von Eckardstein A, Pritchard PH, Albers JJ, Kastelein JJ, Droste C. et al. A molecular defect causing fish eye disease: an amino acid exchange in lecithin-cholesterol acyltransferase (LCAT) leads to the selective loss of alpha- LCAT activity. Proc Natl Acad Sci U S A. 1991;88(11):4855-9. [PMC free article] [PubMed] [Google Scholar]
47. Klein HG, Lohse P, Pritchard PH, Bojanovski D, Schmidt H, Brewer HB Jr. Two different allelic mutations in the lecithin-cholesterol acyltransferase gene associated with the fish eye syndrome Lecithin-cholesterol acyltransferase (Thr123----Ile) and lecithin-cholesterol acyltransferase (Thr347----Met) J Clin Invest. 1992;89(2):499-506. [PMC free article] [PubMed] [Google Scholar]
48. Gigante M, Ranieri E, Cerullo G, Calabresi L, Iolascon A, Assmann G. et al. LCAT deficiency: molecular and phenotypic characterization of an Italian family. J Nephrol. 2006;19(3):375-81. [PubMed] [Google Scholar]

49. Seidel D, Alaupovic P, Furman RH. A lipoprotein characterizing obstructive jaundice I Method for quantitative separation and identification of lipoproteins in jaundiced subjects. J Clin Invest. 1969;48(7):1211-23. [PMC free article] [PubMed] [Google Scholar]

50. Chen C, Applegate K, King WC, Glomset JA, Norum KR, Gjone E. A study of the small spherical high density lipoproteins of patients afflicted with familial lecithin: cholesterol acyltransferase deficiency. J Lipid Res. 1984;25(3):269-82. [PubMed] [Google Scholar]

51. Borysiewicz LK, Soutar AK, Evans DJ, Thompson GR, Rees AJ. Renal failure in familial lecithin: cholesterol acyltransferase deficiency. Q J Med. 1982;51(204):411-26. [PubMed] [Google Scholar]

52. Ohta Y, Yamamoto S, Tsuchida H, Murano S, Saitoh Y, Tohjo S. et al. Nephropathy of familial lecithin-cholesterol acyltransferase deficiency: report of a case. Am J Kidney Dis. 1986;7(1):41-6. [PubMed] [Google Scholar]

53. Holleboom AG, Kuivenhoven JA, van Olden CC, Peter J, Schimmel AW, Levels JH. et al. Proteinuria in early childhood due to familial LCAT deficiency caused by loss of a disulfide bond in lecithin:cholesterol acyl transferase. Atherosclerosis. 2011;216(1):161–5. [PubMed] [Google Scholar]

54. Jahanzad I, Amoueian S, Attaranzadeh A. Familial lecithin-cholesterol acyltransferasedeficiency. ArchIranMed. 2009;12(2):179-81. [PubMed] [Google Scholar]

55. Aranda P, Valdivielso P, Pisciotta L, Garcia I, Garca AAC, Bertolini S. et al. Therapeutic management of a new case of LCAT deficiency with a multifactorial long-term approach based on high doses of angiotensin II receptor blockers (ARBs) Clin Nephrol. 2008;69(3):213-8. [PubMed] [Google Scholar]

56. Miarka P, Idzior-Walus B, Kuzniewski M, Walus-Miarka M, Klupa T, Sulowicz W. Corticosteroid treatment of kidney disease in a patient with familial lecithin-cholesterol acyltransferase deficiency. Clin Exp Nephrol. 2011;15(3):424-9. [PubMed] [Google Scholar]

57. Panescu V, Grignon Y, Hestin D, Rostoker G, Frimat L, Renoult E. et al. Recurrence of lecithin cholesterol acyltransferase deficiency after kidney transplantation. NephrolDialTransplant. 1997;12(11):2430–2. [PubMed] [Google Scholar]

58. Asada S, Kuroda M, Aoyagi Y, Fukaya Y, Tanaka S, Konno S. et al. Ceiling culture-derived proliferative adipocytes retain high adipogenic potential suitable for adipocytes. for use as a vehicle for gene transduction therapy. Am J Physiol Cell

physiol. 2011;301(1):C181-5. [PubMed] [Google Scholar]
59. Bomback AS, Song H, D'Agati VD, Cohen SD, Neal A, Appel GB, Rovin BHA new apolipoprotein E mutation, apoE Las Vegas, in a European-American with lipoprotein glomerulopathy.Nephrol Dial Transplant. 2010 Oct;25(10):3442-6. doi: 10.1093/ndt/gfq389. Epub 2010 Jul 11.PMID: 20624773
60. Saito T, Matsunaga A, Oikawa SImpact of lipoprotein glomerulopathy on the relationship between lipids and renal diseases..Am J Kidney Dis. 2006 Feb;47(2):199-211. doi: 10.1053/j.ajkd.2005.10.017.PMID: 16431249 Review.
61. Zhang B, Liu ZH, Zeng CH, Zheng JM, Chen HP, Zhou H, Li LS. Plasma level and genetic variation of apolipoprotein E in patients with lipoprotein glomerulopathy.Chin Med J (Engl). 2005 Apr 5;118(7):555-60.PMID: 15820086
62. Cheung CY, Chan AO, Chan YH, Lee KC, Chan GP, Lau GT, Shek CC, Chau KF, Li CS. A rare cause of nephrotic syndrome: lipoprotein glomerulopathy.Hong Kong Med J. 2009 Feb;15(1):57-60.PMID: 19197098
63. Diamond JR. Hyperlipidemia of nephrosis: pathophysiologic role in progressive glomerular disease.Am J Med. 1989 Nov;87(5N):25N- 29N.PMID: 2486541 Review.
64. Ting JA, McRae SA, Schwartz D, Barbour SJ, Riazy MLipoprotein Glomerulopathy, First Case Report from Canada.Int J Nephrol Renovasc Dis. 2022 Jun 21;15:207-214. doi: 10.2147/IJNRD.S364890. eCollection 2022.PMID: 35761986 **Free PMC article.**

65. An Updated Review and Meta Analysis of Lipoprotein Glomerulopathy. Li MS, Li Y, Liu Y, Zhou XJ, Zhang H.Front Med (Lausanne). 2022 May 6;9:905007. doi: 10.3389/fmed.2022.905007. eCollection 2022.PMID: 35602473

66. Kalatzis V, Antignac C. Cystinosis: from gene to disease. Nephrol Dial Transplant. 2002;17(11):1883-1886. [PubMed] [Google Scholar]
67. 2. Soliman NA, Elmonem MA, van den Heuvel L, et al. Mutational Spectrum of the CTNS Gene in Egyptian Patients with Nephropathic Cystinosis. JIMD Rep. 2014;14:87-97. [Free PMC Article] [PubMed] [Google Scholar]
68. 3. Ivanova E, De Leo MG, De Matteis MA, Levtchenko E. Cystinosis: clinical presentation, pathogenesis and treatment. Pediatr Endocrinol Rev. 2014;12(1):176-84. [PubMed] [Google Scholar]

69. 4. Soliman AN, El-Baroudy R, Rizk A, et al. Nephropathic Cystinosis in Children: an overlooked disease. Saudi J Kidney Dis Transpl. 2009;20(3):436-

42. [PubMed] [Google Scholar]

70. 5. Pache de Faria Guimaraes L, Seguro AC, Shimizu MH, et al. N-acetyl-cysteine is associated to renal function improvement in patients with nephropathiccystinosis. PediatrNephrol. 2014;29(6):1097-102. [PubMed] [Google Scholar]

71. 6. Al Haggar M. Cystinosis as a lysosomal storage disease with multiple mutant alleles: phenotypic-genotypic correlations. World J Nephrol. 2013;2(4):94-102. [Free PMC Article] [PubMed] [Google Scholar]

72. 7 Gultekingil Keser A, Topaloglu R, Bilginer Y, Besbas N. Long-term endocrinologic complications of cystinosis. Minerva Pediatr. 2014;66(2):123-30. [PubMed] [Google Scholar]

73. 8. Emma F, Nesterova G, Langman C, et al. Nephropathic cystinosis: an international consensus document. Nephrol Dial Transplant. 2014;29(4):87-94. [Free PMC Article] [PubMed] [Google Scholar]

74. 9 Galina Nesterova, William Gahl A. Cystinosis: the evolution of a treatable disease. PediatrNephrol.2013;28(1):51-59. [Free CMC Article] [PubMed] [Google Scholar]

75. 10. Nesterova G, Gahl W. Nephropathic cystinosis: late complications of a multisystemicdisease Pediatr Nephrol.2008;23(6):863- 878. [PubMed] [Google Scholar]

76. 11. Cherqui S. Cysteamine therapy: a treatment for cystinosis, not a cure. Kidney Int. 2012;81(2):127-129. [Free PMC Article] [PubMed] [Google Scholar]

77. 12. Ariceta G, Lara E, Camacho JA, et al. Cysteamine (Cystagon®) adherence in patients with cystinosis in Spain: successful in children and a challenge in adolescents and adults. Nephrol Dial Transplant. 2015;30(3):475-80 [Free PMC Article] [PubMed] [Google Scholar]

78. 13. Gahl WA, Balog JZ, Kleta R. Nephropathic cystinosis in adults: natural history and effects of oral cysteamine therapy. Ann Intern Med. 2007;147(4):242-50 [PubMed] [Google Scholar].

79. 14. Brodin-Sartorius A, Tête M-J, Niaudet P, et al. Cysteamine therapy delays the progression of nephropathic cystinosis in late adolescents and adults. Kidney Int. 2012;81(2):179-189. [PubMed] [Google Scholar]

80. 15. Bertholet-Thomas A, Bacchetta J, Tasic V, et al. Nephropathic Cystinosis - A Gap between Developing and Developed Nations. N Engl J Med. 2014;370(14):1366-7. [PubMed] [Google Scholar]
81. 16. Spicer RA, Clayton PA, McTaggart SJ, Zhang GY, Alexander SI. Patient and graft survival following kidney transplantation in recipients with cystinosis: a cohort study. Am J Kidney Dis. 2015;65(1):172-3. [PubMed] [Google Scholar]
82.. Brodehl J, Hagge W, Gellisen K. Changes in kidney function in cystinosis. I. Inulin, PAH and electrolyte clearance in various stages of the disease. Ann Paediatr. 1965;205:131-54.
83. Baum M. The fanconi syndrome of cystinosis: insights into the pathophysiology. Pediatr Nephrol. 1998;12:492-7. 25.
84. Roth KS, Foreman JW, Segal S. The Fanconi syndrome and mechanisms of tubular transport dysfunction. Kidney Int. 1981;20:705-16. 26.
85. Gaide Chevronnay HP, Janssens V, Van Der Smissen P, N'Kuli F, Nevo N, Guiot Y, Levtchenko E, Marbaix E, Pierreux CE, Cherqui S, Antignac C, Courtoy PJ. Time course of pathogenic and adaptation mechanisms in cystinotic mouse kidneys. J Am Soc Nephrol. 2014;25:1256-69. 27.
86. Wilmer MJ, Schoeber JP, van den Heuvel LP, Levtchenko EN. Cystinosis: practical tools for diagnosis and treatment. Pediatr Nephrol. 2011;26:205-15. 28.
87. O'Regan S, Mongeau JG, Robitaille P. A patient with cystinosis presenting with the features of Bartter syndrome. Acta Paediatr Belg. 1980;33:51-2. 29.
88. Ozkan B, Cayir A, Kosan C, Alp H. Cystinosis presenting with findings of barter syndrome. J Clin Res Pediatr Endocrinol. 2011;3:101-4. 30.
89. Gahl WA, Reed GF, Thoene JG, Schulman JD, Rizzo WB, Jonas AJ. Cysteamine therapy for children with nephropathic cystinosis. N Engl J Med. 1987;316:971-7. 31.
90. Asplin JR. Hyperoxaluric calcium nephrolithiasis. Endocrinol Metab Clin North Am. 2002;31:927-949. [PubMed] [Google Scholar]
91. Milliner DS. The primary hyperoxalurias: an algorithm for diagnosis. Am J Nephrol. 2005;25:154-160 [PubMed] [Google Scholar]
92. Robijn S, Hoppe B, Vervaet BA, D'Haese PC, Verhulst A. Hyperoxaluria: a gut-kidney axis? Kidney Int. 2011;80:1146-1158. [PubMed] [Google Scholar]
93. Arena R, Cahalin LP. Evaluation of cardiorespiratory fitness and respiratory muscle function in the obese population. Prog Cardiovasc Dis. 2014;56:457-464. [PubMed] [Google Scholar]

94. Hoppe B, Langman CB. A United States survey on diagnosis, treatment, and outcome of primary hyperoxaluria. Pediatr Nephrol. 2003;18:986- 991 [PubMed] [Google Scholar]
95. Spasovski G, Beck BB, Blau N, Hoppe B, Tasic V. Late diagnosis of primary hyperoxaluria after failed kidney transplantation. Int Urol Nephrol. 2010;42:825-829. [PubMed] [Google Scholar]
96. Lorenzo V,Torres A, Salido E. Primary hyperoxaluria. Nefrologia. 2014;34:398-412. [PubMed] [Google Scholar]
97. Link YH. Juicing is not all juicy. Am J Med. 2013;126:755- 756 [PubMed] [Google Scholar]
98. 9. Getting JE, Gregoire JR, Phul A, Kasten MJ. Oxalate nephropathy due to 'juicing': case report and review. Am J Med. 2013;126:768- 772 [PubMed] [Google Scholar]
99. Holmes RP, Goodman HO, Assimos DG. Contribution of dietary oxalate to urinary oxalate excretion. Kidney Int. 2001;59:270-276. [PubMed] [Google Scholar]
100. Farinelli MP, Richardson KE. Oxalate synthesis from [14C1]glycollate and [14C1]glyoxylate in the hepatectomized rat. Biochim Biophys Acta. 1983;757:8-14. [PubMed] [Google Scholar]
101. Burchell A. Glycogen storage diseases and the liver. Baillieres Clin Gastroenterol. 1998;12(2):337–54. https://doi.org/10.1016/s0950-3528(98) 90138-5.
102. Chen YT, et al. Renal disease in type I glycogen storage disease. N Engl J Med. 1988;318(1):7-11.https://doi.org/10.1056/nejm198801073180102.
103. Lei KJ, et al. Mutations in the glucose-6-phosphatase gene that cause glycogen storage disease type 1a. Science. 1993;262(5133):580–3. https:// doi.org/10.1126/science.8211187.
104. Kishnani PS, et al. Diagnosis and management of glycogen storage disease type I: a practice guideline of the American College of Medical Genetics and Genomics. Genet Med. 2014;16(11): e1. https://doi.org/10. 1038/gim.2014.128.
105. Rajas F, et al. Lessons from new mouse models of glycogen storage disease type 1a in relation to the time course and organ specifcity of the disease. J Inherit Metab Dis. 2015;38(3):521-7. https://doi.org/10.1007/ s10545-014-9761-0.
106. Wolfsdorf JI, Lafel LM, Crigler JF Jr. Metabolic control and renal dysfunction in type I glycogen storage disease. J Inherit Metab Dis. 1997;20(4):559-68. https://doi.org/10.1023/a:1005346824368.

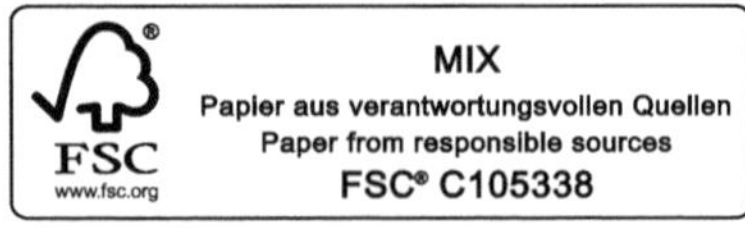

Printed by Books on Demand GmbH, Norderstedt / Germany